T0327506

Atlas of Dermatopathology

Atlas of Dermatopathology

Practical Differential Diagnosis by Clinicopathologic Pattern

Editors

Günter Burg MD

Department of Dermatology
University Hospital Zurich
Zürich
Switzerland

Werner Kempf MD

Department of Dermatology
University Hospital Zurich
Zürich
Switzerland

Heinz Kutzner MD

Dermatopathology Institute
Friedrichshafen
Germany

Co-Editors

Josef Feit MD, PhD

Pathology and Dermatopathology
MDgK plus, Biovendor
Brno
Czech Republic

Laszlo J Karai MD, PhD

Pathology and Dermatopathology
Miami Lakes
FL, USA

WILEY Blackwell

Library of Congress Cataloging-in-Publication Data
Atlas of dermatopathology (Burg)
 Atlas of dermatopathology: practical differential diagnosis by clinicopathologic pattern / editors, Günter Burg, Werner Kempf, Heinz Kutzner ; co-editors, Josef Feit and Laszlo Karai.
   p. ; cm.
 Includes bibliographical references and index.
 ISBN 978-1-118-65831-4 (hardback)
 I. Burg, Günter, editor. II. Kempf, Werner, editor. III. Kutzner, Heinz, editor. IV. Feit, Josef, editor. V. Karai, Laszlo, editor. VI. Title.
 [DNLM: 1. Skin Diseases–pathology–Atlases. 2. Diagnosis, Differential–Atlases. 3. Skin Diseases–diagnosis–Atlases. WR 17]
 RL105
 616.5′075–dc23
                              2015006613

A catalogue record for this book is available from the British Library.

Wiley also publishes its books in a variety of electronic formats. Some content that appears in print may not be available in electronic books.

Set in 8.5/12pt Meridien LT Std by SPi Global, Chennai, India

1 2015

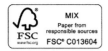

To our families and teachers

Contents

Preface

This atlas is addressed to pathologists and dermatologists who intend to become familiar with a practical approach to dermatopathology.

The structure of the book and of its chapters follows a basic approach to morphology. In histomorphology, as in clinical (macro-)morphology, the first step is to identify the localization of the pathological changes which is mostly done at scanning magnification; the second step includes assessing the distribution or pattern of pathologic elements at higher magnification and finally to search for the pathognomic elements – the so-called diagnostic clues.

It is like approaching a painting. In one of the almost 50 cabinets of the Alte Pinakothek in Munich, German paintings of the 14th–17th century are displayed (step 1). Among them one can detect a wonderful painting by Albrecht Altdorfer (1529) (step 2). Looking more closely one will discover between the many details Darius of Persia in flight and Alexander of Greece pursuing him (step 3). This is the clue for the "diagnosis," telling us that the Battle of Issus (333 BC), occident against orient, is the main theme of the painting.

Looking at a microscopic slide, our brain is following the same approach of overall orientation, identifying a prototypic pattern and finding the essential clue(s) for the diagnosis.

Therefore, in this book histo- and cytomorphologic elements should give guidance rather than any pathogenetic parameters we may have in our minds. Starting with the cornified layer of the epidermis, the chapters follow the pathological findings in the various levels of the epidermis, dermis and subcutaneous fat tissue and describe and display prototypes of diagnoses, their variants and the differential diagnoses, which may simulate the prototype. Each diagnosis is shown by its clinical appearance (Cl:) and by its histomorphology (Hi:) at

The Battle of Alexander at Issus 333 BC by Albrecht Altdorfer.
(bpk/Bayerische Staatsgemäldesammlung, München)

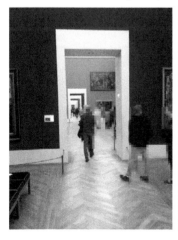 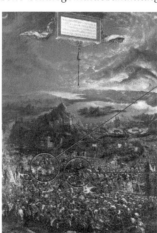 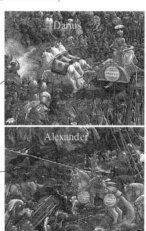

scanning magnification and at high power magnification, pointing to special clues.

Descriptions in *italic* are not displayed as pictures in the same chapter, but may be demonstrated in another one.

Many of the histologic images shown are taken from the *Hypertext Atlas of Dermatopathology* (www.atlases.muni.cz).[1]

References are not comprehensive, but may be of some help for getting more detailed information.

---

[1] *Hypertext Atlas of Dermatopathology* Josef Feit, Hana Jedličková, Zdeněk Vlašín, Günter Burg, Werner Kempf, Leo Schärer, Luděk Matyska (www.atlases.muni.cz)

Abbreviations

Cl	Clinical features		**HPF**	High power field
CNS	Central nervous system		**PAS**	Periodic acid-Schiff
DIF	Direct Immunofluorescence		**PCR**	Polymerase chain reaction
Hi	Histological features			

Dermatopathology

Text-Atlas for Practical Differential Diagnosis of Clinicopathologic Pattern of Inflammatory Skin Diseases

Editors: Günter Burg, Werner Kempf, Heinz Kutzner

Co-Editors: Josef Feit and Laszlo Karai

Atlas of Dermatopathology: Practical Differential Diagnosis by Clinicopathologic Pattern, First Edition.
Edited by Günter Burg MD, Werner Kempf MD, and Heinz Kutzner MD. Co-Editors: Josef Feit MD, and Laszlo Karai MD.
© 2015 John Wiley & Sons, Ltd. Published 2015 by John Wiley & Sons, Ltd.

Introduction

Some basic terms in dermatohistology

Horny layer

Orthokeratosis: Basket weave stratum corneum

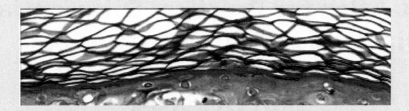

Hyperkeratosis: Thickened stratum corneum

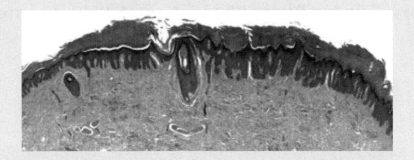

Parakeratosis: Remnants of nuclei in stratum corneum

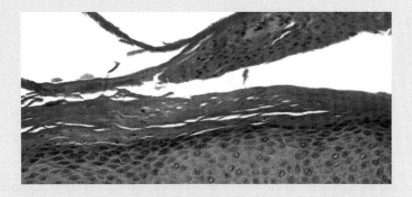

Epidermis

Atrophy

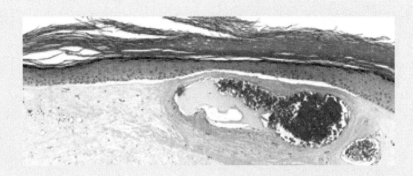

Acanthosis

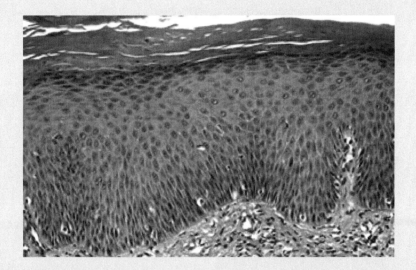

Papillomatosis

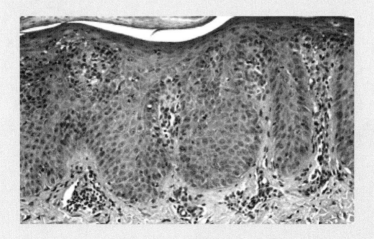

INTRODUCTION

Hypergranulomatosis

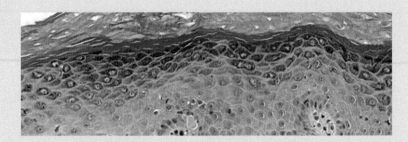

Spongiosis

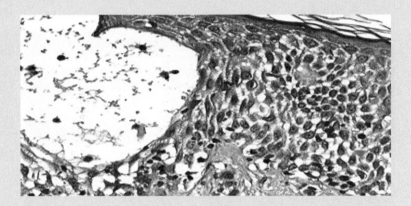

Acantholysis

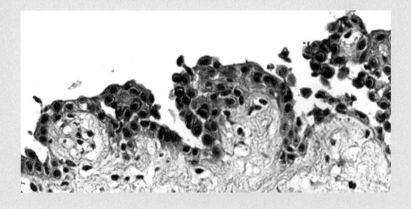

Ballooning

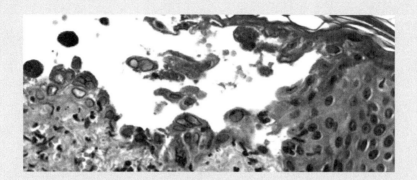

Dyskeratosis(*)

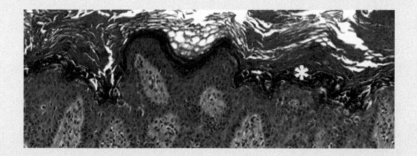

Necrotic keratinocytes

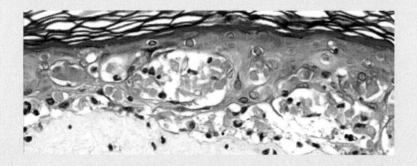

Interface

Interface dermatitis

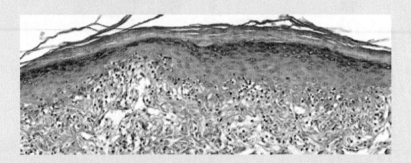

Subepidermal blistering

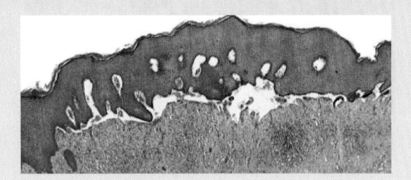

Subepidermal edema

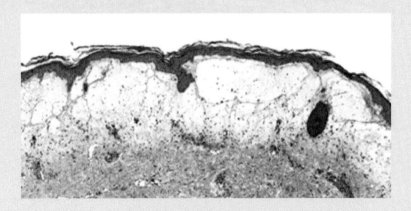

Dermis

Fibrosis

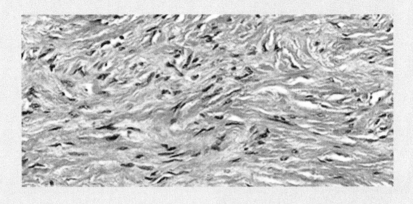

Sclerosis

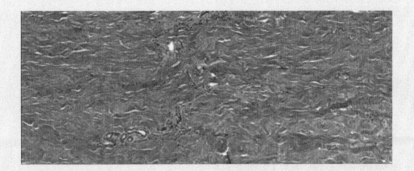

Elastosis, actinic

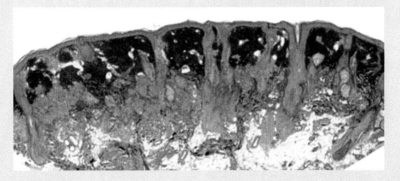

Elastica stain

INTRODUCTION

Vasculitis

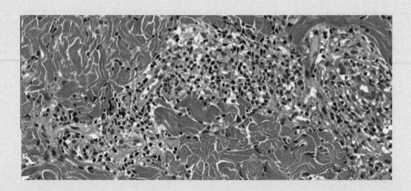

Calcification (vessel wall)

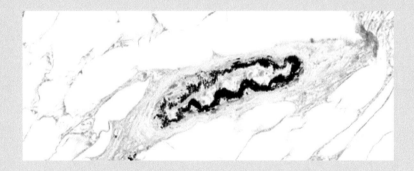

Langhans giant cells with *acid fast bacilli* (inset)

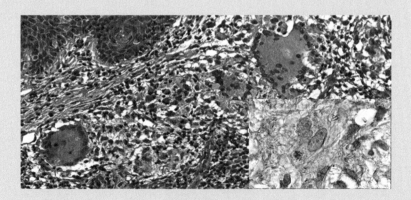

Foreign body giant cells

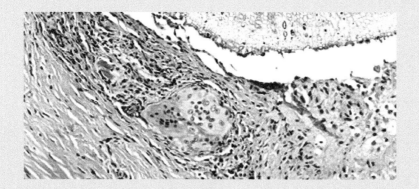

Touton giant cells

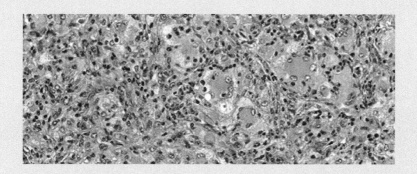

Clinicopathologic Correlation

When considering clinicopathologic correlations in approaching a diagnosis there basically are four scenarios, in which the diagnostic impact of histopathology may be high, moderate, low or none.

1. High diagnostic impact of histology, when the clinical presentations are almost identical

Psoriasis (left) vs seborrheic dermatitis (right)

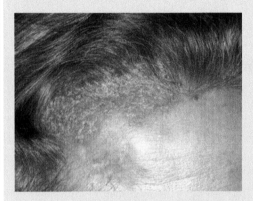 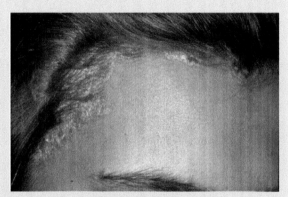

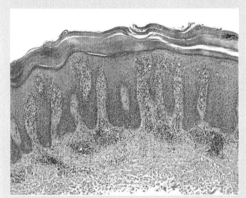 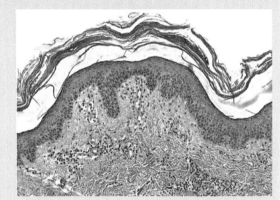

Psoriasiform acanthosis

Free floating parakeratotic scale without psoriasiform acanthosis

Urticaria (left) vs Sweet's syndrome (right)

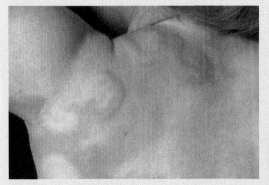 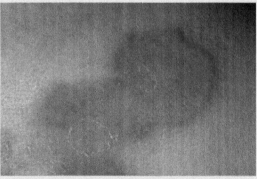

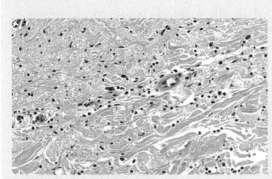

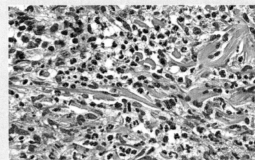

Sparse granulocytic infiltrate

Densely packed sheets of neutrophils

Lichen planus (left) vs lichen sclerosus et atrophicus (right)

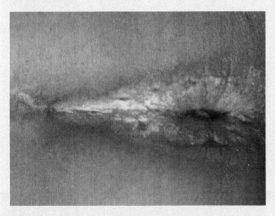

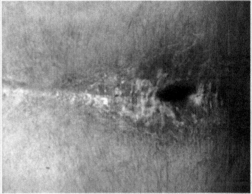

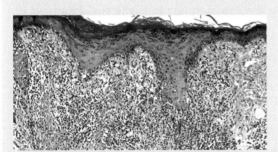

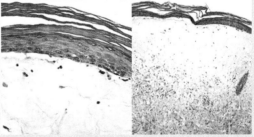

Sawtooth pattern with hypergranulosis and lichenoid interface dermatitis

Tricolore pattern with red epidermis, white sclerosis, and blue band-like infiltrate.

2. Moderate diagnostic impact of histology, when the histology is just confirmation of the clinical diagnosis and is not mandatory as such

Nummular dermatitis (left) vs fungal infection (tinea) (right)

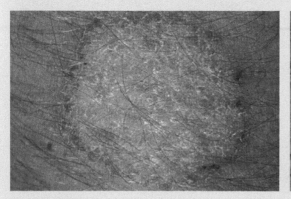
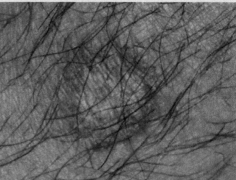

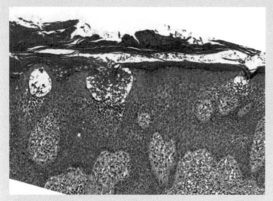
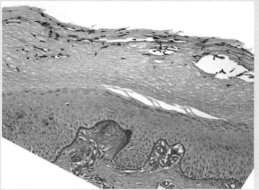

Scale crust without fungal organisms.   Hyphae and spores within cornified layer.

3. Low diagnostic impact of histology, when the clinician has to make the diagnosis based on the clinical presentation

Transient acantholytic dermatosis (Grover's disease) (left) vs benign chronic familial pemphigus (Hailey-Hailey disease) (right)

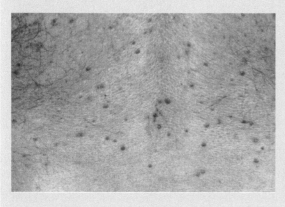
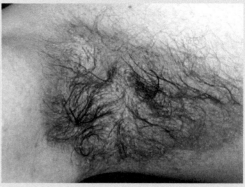

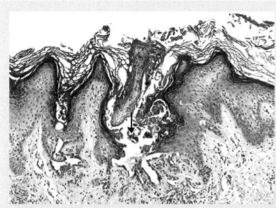

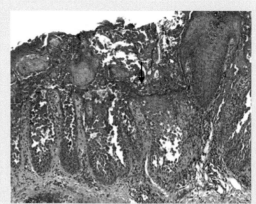

Focal acantholytic dyskeratosis (arrow)   Transepidermal acantholysis (arrow)

Systemic diffuse scleroderma (left) vs circumscribed scleroderma (morphea) (right)

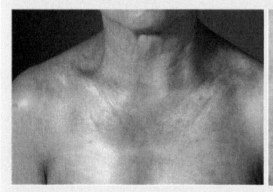

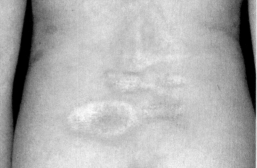

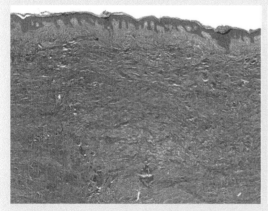

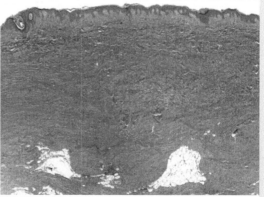

INTRODUCTION

Dermatomyositis (left) vs acute systemic lupus erythematosus (right)

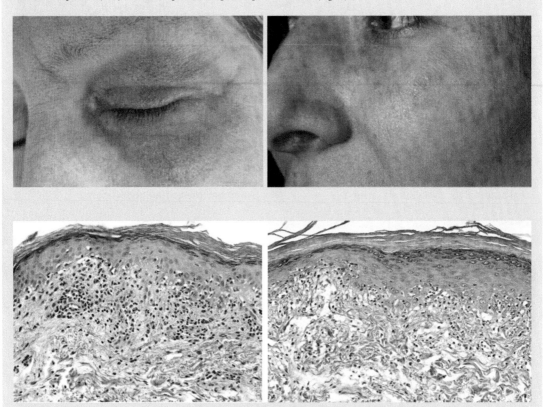

Denser infiltrate.   Less round cell infiltrate, more mucin deposits.

4. Little or no diagnostic impact of histology, when neither the clinical nor the histological presentation allows a definite diagnosis, which often is revealed only by the clinical course or the therapeutic susceptibility

Pseudolymphoma (left) vs cutaneous B-cell lymphoma (right)

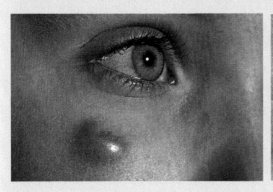
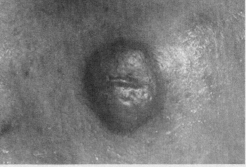

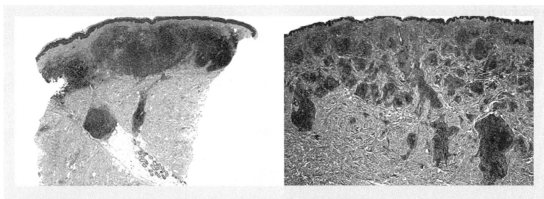

Similar pattern and immunophenotype in both lymphatic infiltrates.

The Diagnostic Puzzle

Even though apart from a thorough history, clinical presentation and histomorphology are the basic elements in reaching a proper diagnosis, additional investigations like immunophenotyping, genotyping and molecular techniques in conjunction with laboratory investigations sometimes are very helpful in completing a complex puzzle by "rearrangements" of various facts.

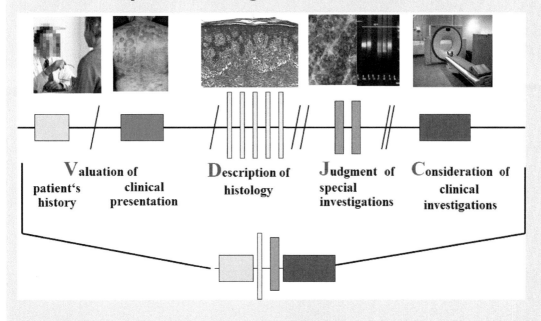

INTRODUCTION

Helpful links

For more information on common skin diseases you can register and login free of charge at DOIT (Dermatology Online with Interactive Technology; www.cyberderm.net).

For guidance through the program have a look on YouTube: https://www.youtube.com/watch?v=3ekhor35w0w&feature=emm-upload_owner#action=share.

A Collection of high resolution histological images are presented free of charge in the Hypertext Atlas of Dermatopathology (www.atlases.muni.cz).

CHAPTER 1

Horny Layer

CHAPTER MENU

Reduced granular layer
Prominent granular layer

Atlas of Dermatopathology: Practical Differential Diagnosis by Clinicopathologic Pattern, First Edition.
Edited by Günter Burg MD, Werner Kempf MD, and Heinz Kutzner MD. Co-Editors: Josef Feit MD, and Laszlo Karai MD.
© 2015 John Wiley & Sons, Ltd. Published 2015 by John Wiley & Sons, Ltd.

HORNY LAYER

PROTOTYPE: Ichthyosis vulgaris

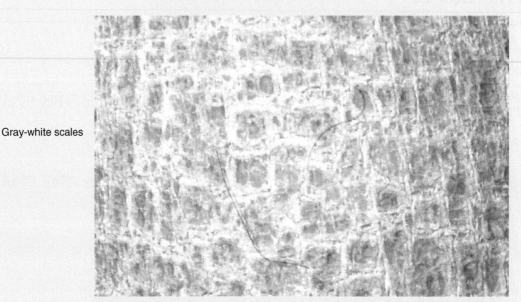

Gray-white scales

CI: Starts in first year of life, dry rough scaly skin, gray-white scales are shed, symmetrical sparing of flexural areas, hyperlinear palms and soles, often atopic dermatitis (50%).

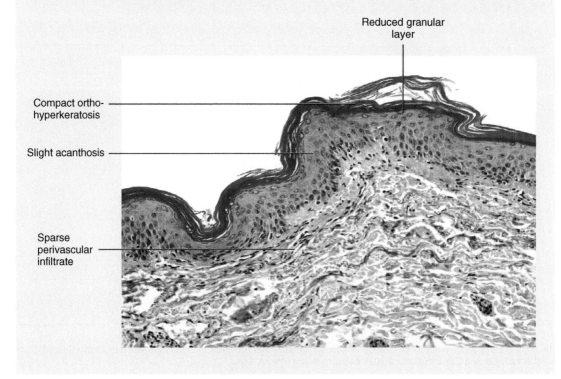

Reduced granular layer

Compact ortho-hyperkeratosis

Slight acanthosis

Sparse perivascular infiltrate

Ichthyosis vulgaris

Compact ortho-
hyperkeratosis

Sparse
perivascular
infiltrate

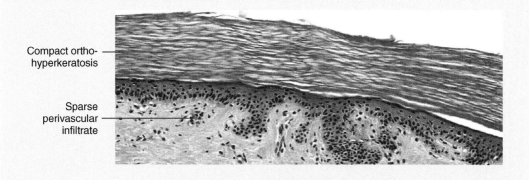

Reduced
granular layer

Slight
acanthosis

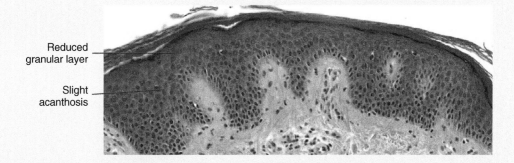

Follicular dilatation
and hyperkeratosis

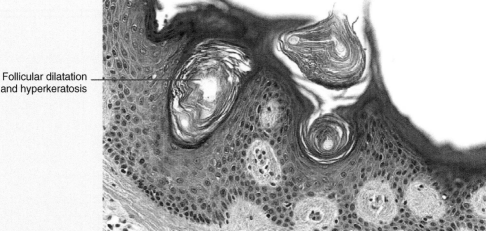

Hi: Compact orthohyperkeratosis, granular layer reduced or absent, lack of parakeratosis, follicular dilatation and hyperkeratosis. Epidermis usually normal, sometimes acanthotic or atrophic. No or sparse perivascular infiltrate in the papillary dermis.

VARIANTS: **Acquired ichthyosis vulgaris**

Histology is identical to ichthyosis vulgaris.

DIFFERENTIAL DIAGNOSIS: **Ichthyosis hystrix**

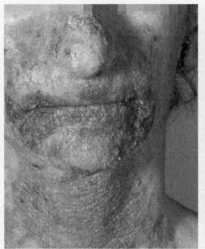
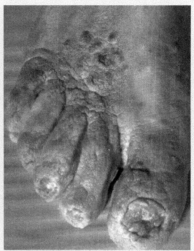

Massive
hyperkeratosis

Cl: Massive, dark, sometimes spiny hyperkeratosis. Various genetic forms exist.
Flexures, palms and soles are involved.

Papillomatosis   Perinuclear vacuolization

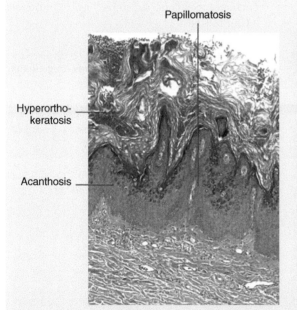
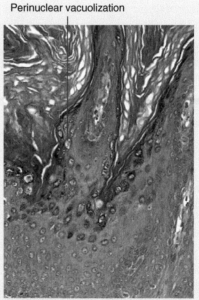

Hyperortho-
keratosis

Acanthosis

Hi: Mild hyperorthokeratosis, acanthosis, papillomatosis, elongation of rete
ridges. Perinuclear vacuolization of granular and spinous layer keratinocytes,
presenting epidermolytic features.

Other Diagnosis

Refsum syndrome (heredopathia atactica polyneuritiformis): Vacuolization of basal and suprabasal keratinocytes (accumulation of phytanic acid; Sudan red stain)

X-linked dominant ichthyosis (Harlequin ichthyosis): Clinical features similar to ichthyosis vulgaris, but flexures are involved, undescended testes in 30%. Vacuolization of basal and suprabasal keratinocytes (accumulation of phytanic acid; Sudan red stain)

Lamellar ichthyosis: Genetically heterogeneous disorder, usually present at birth presenting as collodion baby in case of generalized involvement. Erythrodermic and non-erythrodermic forms. Transglutaminase-deficiency in most forms. Histology shows mild to moderate hyperorthokeratosis, stratum granulosum normal or broadened, acanthosis, papillomatosis

Bullous, epidermolytic ichthyosis (bullous form of erythrodermia ichthyosiformis congenitalis): Erythroderma at birth with diffuse blistering and erosions, like burned. Histologically the most striking feature is acanthokeratolysis with epidermal thickening leading to superficial blister formation. Tonofilaments can be seen as dark clumps in a shell-like arrangement around the nucleus

Syndromes of ichthyosis and trichothiodystrophy (Tay syndrome): Additional clinical symptoms and biochemical findings.

References

de Berker, D., W. A. Branford, S. Soucek, and L. Michaels (1993). "Fatal keratitis ichthyosis and deafness syndrome (KIDS). Aural, ocular, and cutaneous histopathology." *Am J Dermatopathol* **15**(1): 64–9.

de Wolf, K., J. M. Gourdain, G. D. Dobbeleer, and M. Song (1995). "A particular subtype of ichthyosis congenita type III. Clinical, light, and electron microscopic features." *Am J Dermatopathol* **17**(6): 606–11.

Frenk, E. and B. Mevorah (1977). "The keratinization disorder in collodion babies evolving into lamellar ichthyosis. Its possible relevance for determining the primary defect in lamellar ichthyosis." *J Cutan Pathol* **4**(6): 329–37.

Hoang, M. P., K. R. Carder, A. G. Pandya, and M. J. Bennett (2004). "Ichthyosis and keratotic follicular plugs containing dystrophic calcification in newborns: distinctive histopathologic features of x-linked dominant chondrodysplasia punctata (Conradi-Hunermann-Happle syndrome)." *Am J Dermatopathol* **26**(1): 53–8.

Nabai, H. and A. H. Mehregan (1979). "Ichthyosis linearis circumflexa." *J Cutan Pathol* **6**(2): 148–9.

Niemi, K. M. and L. Kanerva (1989). "Ichthyosis with laminated membrane structures." *Am J Dermatopathol* **11**(2): 149–56.

Niemi, K. M., K. Kuokkanen, L. Kanerva, and J. Ignatius (1993). "Recessive ichthyosis congenita type IV." *Am J Dermatopathol* **15**(3): 224–8.

Okulicz, J. F. and R. A. Schwartz (2003). "Hereditary and acquired ichthyosis vulgaris." *Int J Dermatol* **42**(2): 95–8.

Sandler, B. and K. Hashimoto (1998). "Collodion baby and lamellar ichthyosis." *J Cutan Pathol* **25**(2): 116–21.

PROTOTYPE: Lamellar ichthyosis

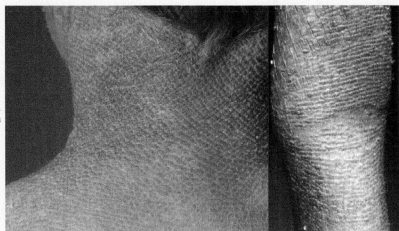

Lamellar ichthyosis. Neck and cubital area

Cl: Genetically heterogeneous disorder, usually manifest at birth presenting as collodion baby in case of generalized involvement. Erythrodermic and non-erythrodermic forms. Transglutaminase deficiency in most forms.

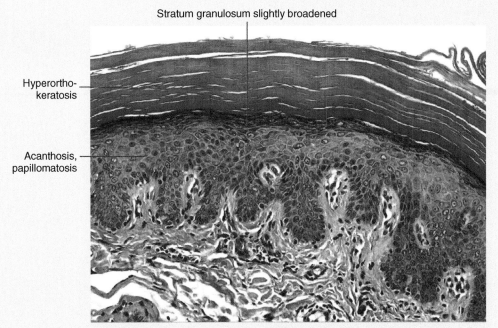

Stratum granulosum slightly broadened

Hyperortho-keratosis

Acanthosis, papillomatosis

Hi: Mild to moderate hyperorthokeratosis, stratum granulosum normal or broadened, acanthosis, papillomatosis.

DIFFERENTIAL DIAGNOSIS: Congenital ichthyosis group X-linked dominant ichthyosis (Harlequin ichthyosis)

Cl: Similar to ichthyosis vulgaris, but flexures are involved, undescended testes in 30%.

Hi: Vacuolization of basal and suprabasal keratinocytes (accumulation of phytanic acid; Sudan red stain).

HORNY LAYER

DIFFERENTIAL DIAGNOSIS: X-linked recessive ichthyosis

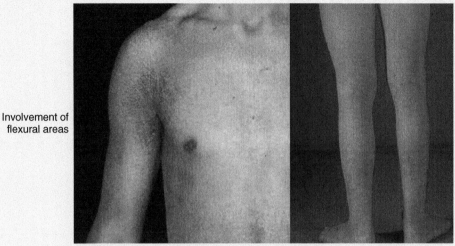

Involvement of flexural areas

Cl: Starts in the first week of life with fine scales and mild erythema, aggravating after a few months. Brown scales giving a dirty appearance cover the whole integument, without sparing of flexural areas.

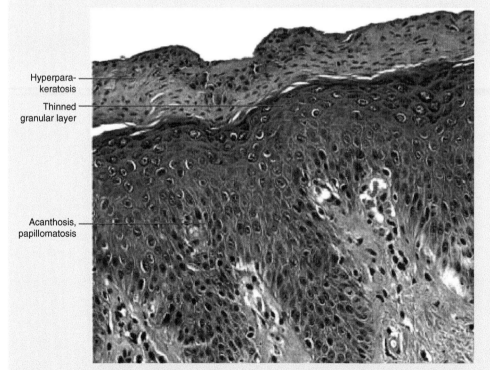

Hyperpara-keratosis

Thinned granular layer

Acanthosis, papillomatosis

Hi: Marked hyperkeratosis, thickened or normal and sometimes thinned granular layer, spinous layer variably acanthotic and papillomatous, mild to marked perivascular infiltrate in the papillary dermis.

HORNY LAYER

DIFFERENTIAL DIAGNOSIS: Bullous epidermolytic ichthyosis (bullous form of congenital ichthyosiform erythroderma)

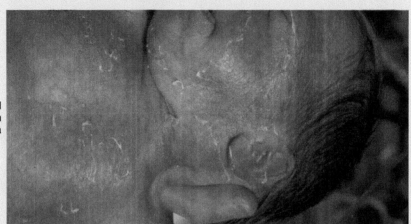

Congenital ichthyosiform erythroderma

CI: Erythroderma at birth with diffuse blistering and erosions, as if burned.

Epidermolytic changes

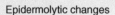
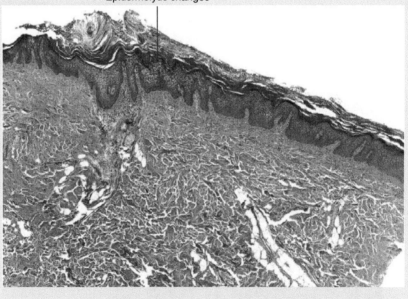

Bullous epidermolytic ichthyosis

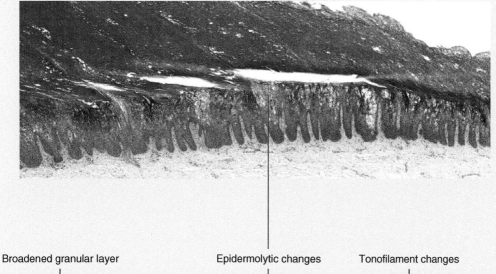

Broadened granular layer   Epidermolytic changes   Tonofilament changes

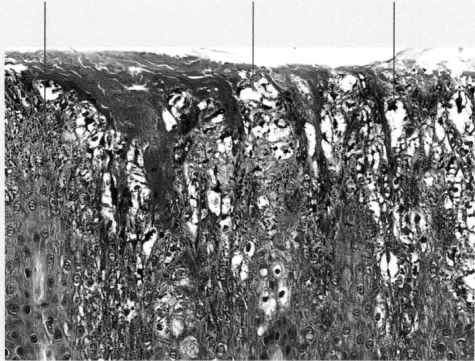

Hi: Epidermolytic changes in the upper part of the spinous and the broadened granular layer, which may lead to superficial blister formation. Tonofilaments can be seen as dark clumps in a shell-like arrangement around the nucleus.

Ichthyosis and deafness syndromes: *Additional clinical symptoms and biochemical findings*

- *Ichthyosis and deafness syndromes*
  - *Hystrix-like ichthyosis with deafness (HID)*
  - *Keratitis, ichthyosis-like hyperkeratosis and deafness (KID)*
- *Ichthyosis hystrix Curth-Macklin: epidermolytic changes without bullae*
- *Erythrodermia congenitalis ichthyosiformis*
- *Neutral lipid storage disease with ichthyosiform erythroderma (Dorfman syndrome): foamy cytoplasm of keratinocytes in the basal and the granular layer*

Erythrokeratoderma variabilis, various forms: *Migratory erythema and/or persistent hyperkeratotic plaques. Orthohyperkeratosis over a normal granular layer, acanthosis and papillomatosis. Perivascular lymphocytic infiltrate of variable intensity in the upper dermis*

DIFFERENTIAL DIAGNOSIS: Other Skin Diseases

- *Acanthosis nigricans: confined to flexural areas. Hyperpigmentation of epidermal basal layer*
- *Epidermal nevus* (*see* Chapter 2, Pruriginous, page 47) *circumscribed lesion with acanthosis and hyperkeratosis*
- *Palmoplantar keratodermas: confined to palmoplantar areas*
- *Chronic eczema (lichen simplex chronicus)* (*see* Chapter 2, Chronic, page 36) *foci of parakeratosis, perivascular lymphocytic infiltrate in the upper dermis*
- *Pityriasis rubra pilaris* (*see* Chapter 2, psoriasiform, page 56): *Horizontally and vertically alternating ortho- and hyperparakeratosis (checkerboard sign). Subtle perivascular infiltrate, clinically nappes claires*
- *Clavus* (*see* Chapter 2, Pruriginous, page 46): *Circumscribed lesion with acanthosis and hyperkeratosis. No inflammation*

HORNY LAYER

References

Hoang, M. P., K. R. Carder, *et al.* (2004). "Ichthyosis and keratotic follicular plugs containing dystrophic calcification in newborns: distinctive histopathologic features of x-linked dominant chondrodysplasia punctata (Conradi-Hunermann-Happle syndrome)." *Am J Dermatopathol* **26**(1): 53–8.

CHAPTER 2

Epidermis

<table>
<tr><td colspan="2">CHAPTER MENU</td></tr>
<tr><td>Eczematous</td><td>Pustular</td></tr>
<tr><td> Acute</td><td>Degenerative</td></tr>
<tr><td> Subacute</td><td> Necrotic</td></tr>
<tr><td> Chronic</td><td> Ballooning</td></tr>
<tr><td> Pruriginous</td><td> Koilocytic</td></tr>
<tr><td>Psoriasiform</td><td>Atrophic</td></tr>
<tr><td>Bullous, acantholytic</td><td></td></tr>
</table>

Atlas of Dermatopathology: Practical Differential Diagnosis by Clinicopathologic Pattern, First Edition.
Edited by Günter Burg MD, Werner Kempf MD, and Heinz Kutzner MD. Co-Editors: Josef Feit MD, and Laszlo Karai MD.
© 2015 John Wiley & Sons, Ltd. Published 2015 by John Wiley & Sons, Ltd.

EPIDERMIS

PROTOTYPE: Acute (contact) dermatitis

Erythema,
papules and
vesicles

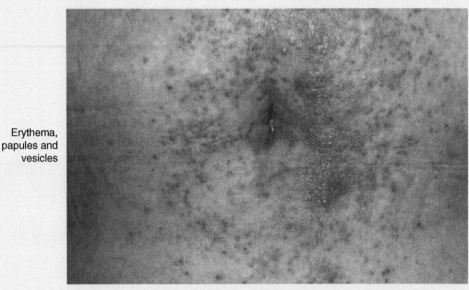

Cl: Erythema, vesicles and crust formation in a fairly circumscribed area.

Spongiotic
vesicles

Acanthosis

Inflammatory
infiltrate

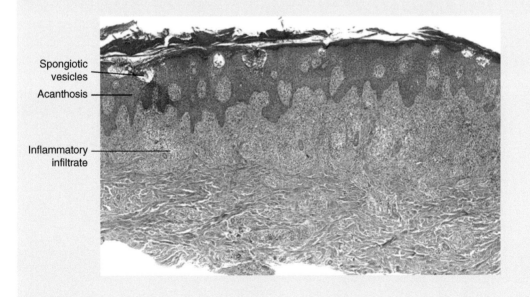

Acute (contact) dermatitis

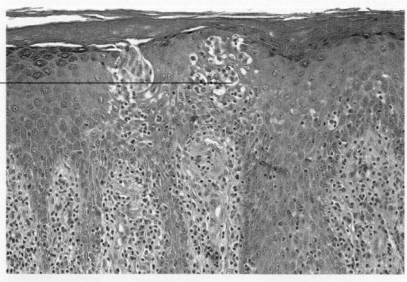

Spongiosis and
accumulation of
Langerhans cells

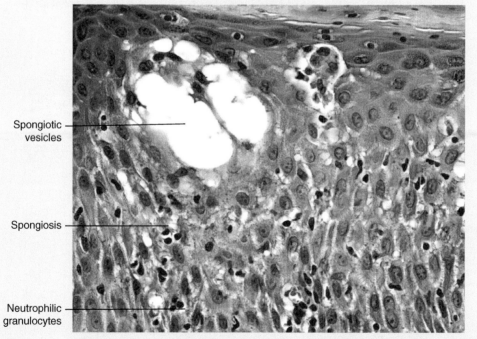

Spongiotic
vesicles

Spongiosis

Neutrophilic
granulocytes

Hi: Spongiosis, acanthosis of variable degree and hyperparakeratosis
of variable degree depending on the evolutionary stage, diffuse and
perivascular predominantly lymphocytic infiltrate with a few eosinophils or
neutrophils, edema of the papillary dermis.

EPIDERMIS

VARIANT: Dyshidrotic eczema

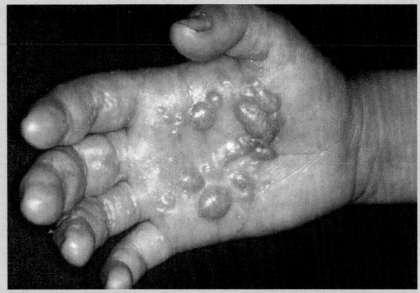

Tense blisters
on the palm

Cl: Small vesicles or larger blisters (pompholyx) on palms and soles.

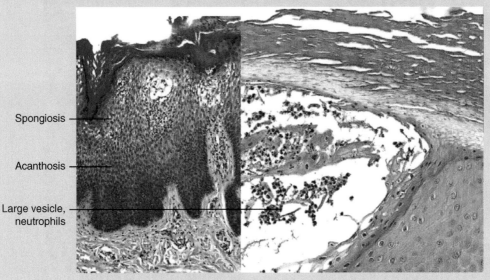

Spongiosis

Acanthosis

Large vesicle,
neutrophils

Hi: Spongiotic vesicles.

Acute toxic contact dermatitis: *necrotic keratinocytes, admixture of neutrophils.*
Acute allergic contact dermatitis: *prominent number of eosinophils.*

DIFFERENTIAL DIAGNOSIS: **Phototoxic and photoallergic dermatitis**

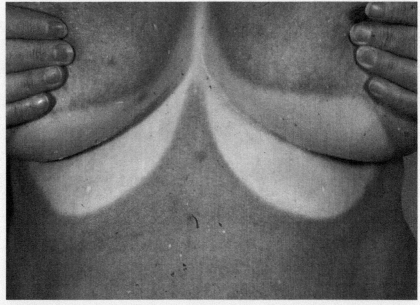

Erythema in
sunlight
exposed areas

Cl: Erythema, vesicles or blisters in sun exposed areas with sharp (toxic) or fairly sharp (allergic) demarcation.

Necrotic
keratinocytes:
«Sunburn cells»

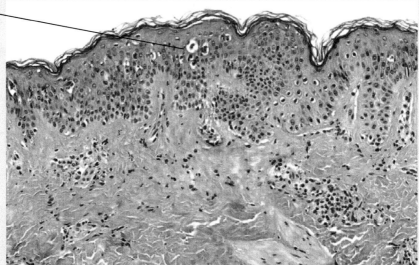

Phototoxic and photoallergic dermatitis

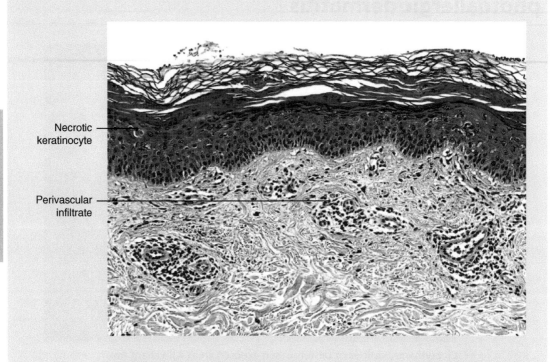

Necrotic
keratinocyte

Perivascular
infiltrate

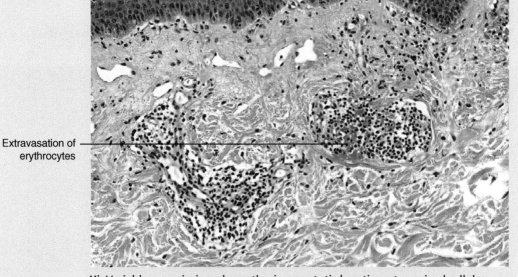

Extravasation of
erythrocytes

Hi: Variable spongiosis and acanthosis, apoptotic keratinocytes, mixed cellular infiltrate, composed of lymphocytes, eosinophils, few neutrophils; extravasation of erythrocytes; dermal edema in the upper dermis.

DIFFERENTIAL DIAGNOSIS: **Polymorphous light eruption**

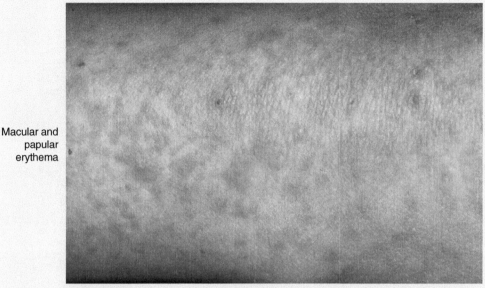

Macular and papular erythema

Cl: Even though PLE is a monomorphous eruption in the affected individual, there are many different (polymorphous) clinical manifestations between individual patients, ranging from erythematous to papular or papulovesicular lesions, which appear exclusively in sun exposed areas.

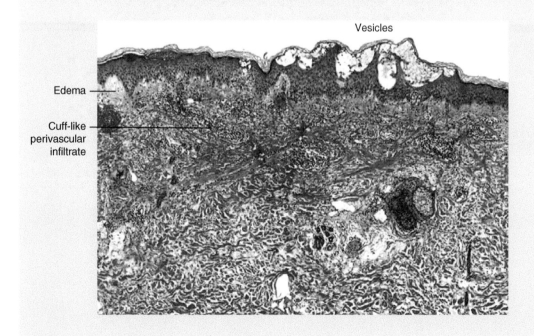

Vesicles

Edema

Cuff-like perivascular infiltrate

Polymorphous light eruption

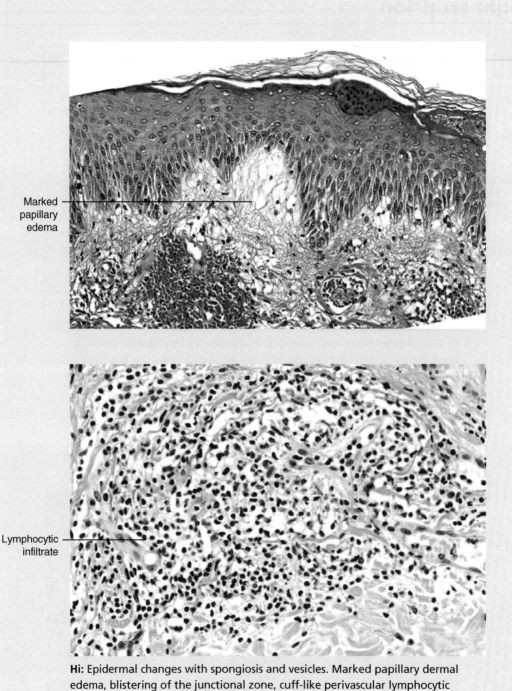

Marked papillary edema

Lymphocytic infiltrate

Hi: Epidermal changes with spongiosis and vesicles. Marked papillary dermal edema, blistering of the junctional zone, cuff-like perivascular lymphocytic infiltrates with eosinophils.

DIFFERENTIAL DIAGNOSIS: **Miliaria cristallina**

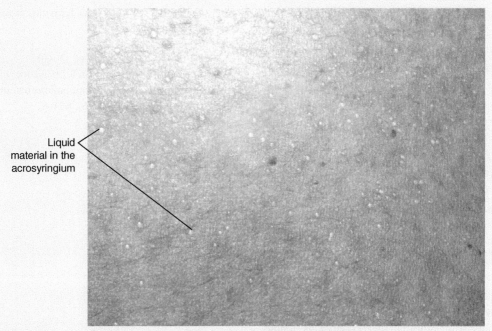

Liquid material in the acrosyringium

Cl: Erythema with crystalline exsudate in the follicular ostia.

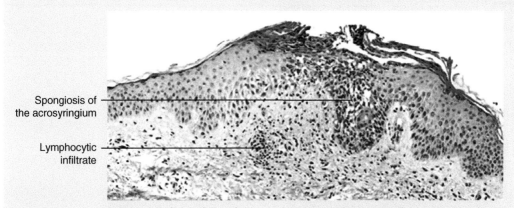

Spongiosis of the acrosyringium

Lymphocytic infiltrate

Hi: Spongiosis involving the acrosyringium. Miliaria cristallina: subcorneal vesicle, neutrophils. Miliaria rubra: spongiosis of the upper half of the acrosyringium, lymphocytic infiltrate around sweat gland ducts in the papillary dermis.

Other Diagnosis

Acute nummular dermatitis: Intracorneal inclusions of serum ("wet" stratum corneum), crust formation, intraepidermal vesicles, neutrophils.

Id-reaction: Clinical context, admixture of eosinophils, focal epidermal changes.

Infestation: Numerous eosinophils, occasionally identifiable organisms, such as scabies or parts of organisms.

Pemphigus vulgaris, prebullous stage: Spongiosis, exocytosis of eosinophils (so-called eosinophilic spongiosis); DIF: intercellular intraepidermal deposits of IgG and C3.

Bullous Pemphigoid: Prebullous stage: spongiosis, exocytosis of eosinophils; DIF: linear deposits of IgG and C3 at the junctional zone.

Cutaneous T-cell lymphoma (spongiotic form): Nuclear atypia and lining-up of lymphocytes at the junctional zone and formation of Pautrier microabscesses.

Incontinentia pigmenti (early vesicular stage): Eosinophilic spongiosis, whorls of necrotic keratinocytes.

Comments

In patients with urticarial and eczematous lesions, which cannot be explained by another cause (contact allergy, atopic dermatitis, eczematous drug eruption), a prebullous phase of pemphigus vulgaris and bullous pemphigoid should be considered as a differential diagnosis. In such patients direct immunofluorescence or immunohistochemical detection of C3d in formalin-fixed biopsies of bullous pemphigoid will be diagnostically very helpful to identify the underlying disease.

References

Aydin, O., B. Engin, O. Oguz, *et al.* (2008). "Non-pustular palmoplantar psoriasis: is histologic differentiation from eczematous dermatitis possible?" *J Cutan Pathol* **35**(2): 169–73.

Pfaltz, K., K. Mertz, C. Rose, *et al.* (2010). "C3d immunohistochemistry on formalin-fixed tissue is a valuable tool in the diagnosis of bullous pemphigoid of the skin." *J Cutan Pathol* **37**(6): 654–8.

PROTOTYPE: **Nummular dermatitis**

Nummular
lesions with
erythema and
desquamation

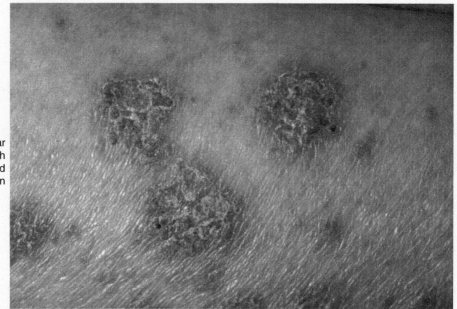

Cl: Nummular (coin-shaped), exsudative patches and plaques, often with crusts.

Parahyperkeratosis

Intracorneal
serum
inclusions

Spongiotic
vesicles

Acanthosis

Lymphocytic
infiltrate

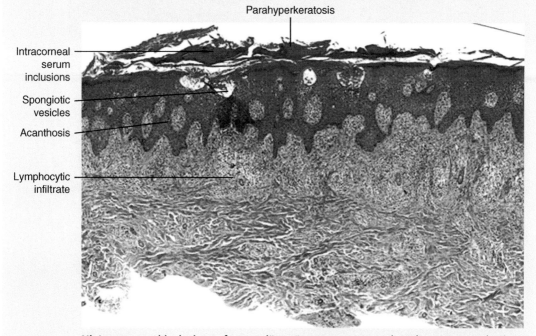

Hi: Intracorneal inclusions of serum ("wet" stratum corneum); scale-crust, acanthosis, hyperparakeratosis, intraepidermal vesicles, diffuse and perivascular infiltrate of lymphocytes and eosinophils and/or neutrophils.

EPIDERMIS

Nummular dermatitis

Exsudate and crust —

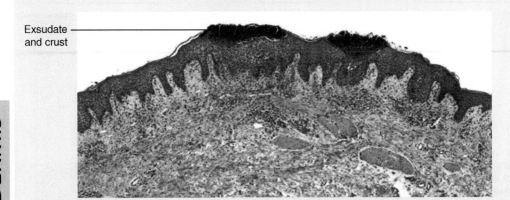

Crust —

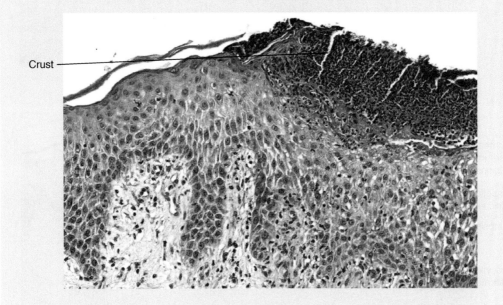

Nummular dermatitis

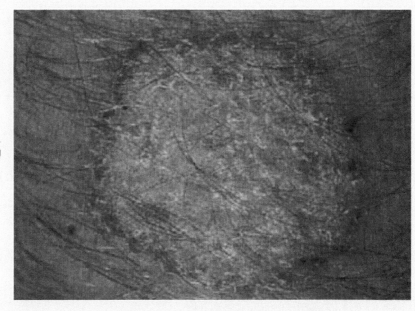

Nummular lesion.
Erythema, scaling

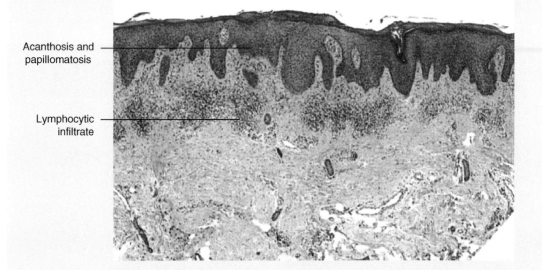

Acanthosis and
papillomatosis

Lymphocytic
infiltrate

EPIDERMIS

DIFFERENTIAL DIAGNOSIS: Pityriasis rosea

Erythematous
patches,
slight scaling

Collarette

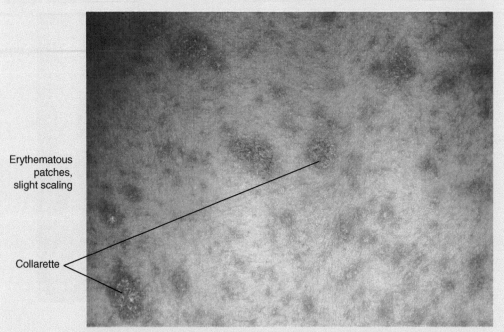

Cl: Disseminated erythematous patches with superficial scaling; process starts with a single oval herald patch.

Patchy hyperkeratosis   Patchy superficial infiltrate

Acanthosis

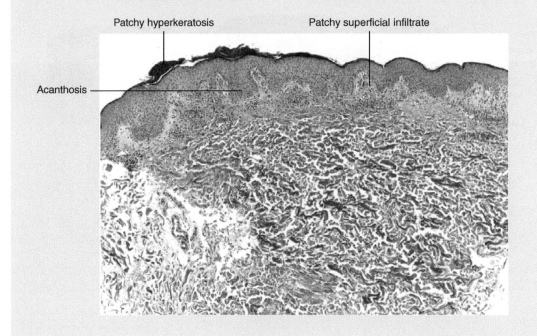

Pityriasis rosea

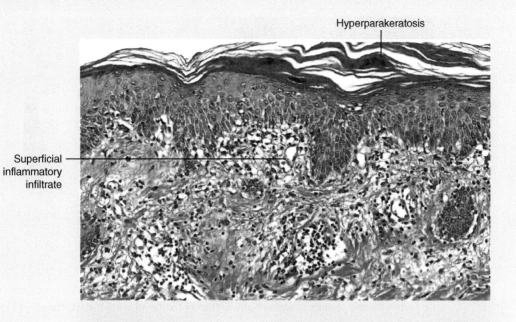

Hyperparakeratosis

Superficial inflammatory infiltrate

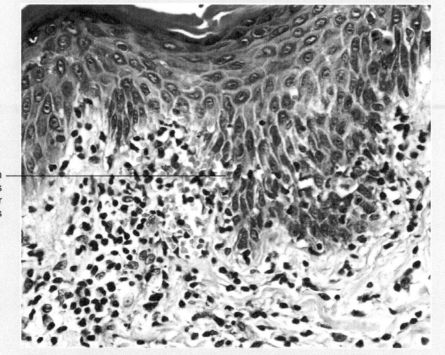

Erythrocytes in the epidermis and in the upper dermis

Hi: Focal hyperparakeratosis, slight spongiosis, lymphocytic infiltrate in the upper dermis, intraepidermal erythrocytes.

DIFFERENTIAL DIAGNOSIS: **Seborrheic dermatitis**

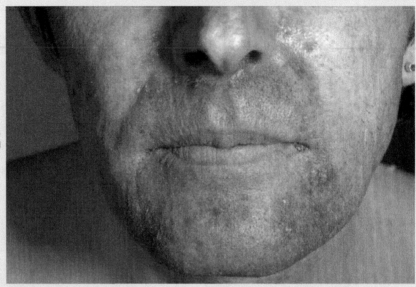

Erythema,
slight scaling

Cl: Erythema and scaling, preferentially in the centro-facial area, breast, scalp.

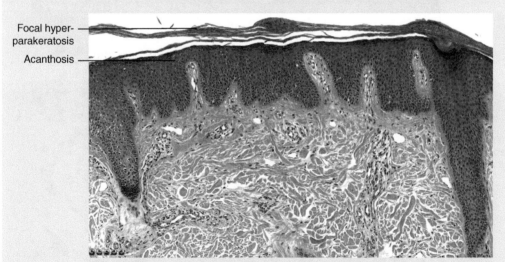

Focal hyper-
parakeratosis

Acanthosis

Hi: Psoriasiform acanthosis and hyperparakeratosis overlying hair follicle ostia, exocytosis of neutrophils.

DIFFERENTIAL DIAGNOSIS: Erythema annulare centrifugum

Annular lesions

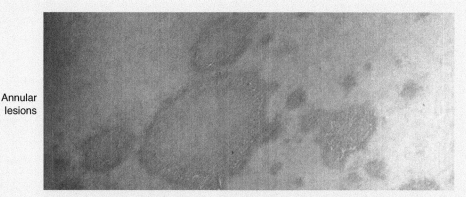

Cl: Centrifugal erythematous rings with slight elevation, scaling and central regression.

Crust from scratching

Cuff-like perivascular infiltrate

Hyperparakeratosis

Slight acanthosis

Perivascular infiltrate

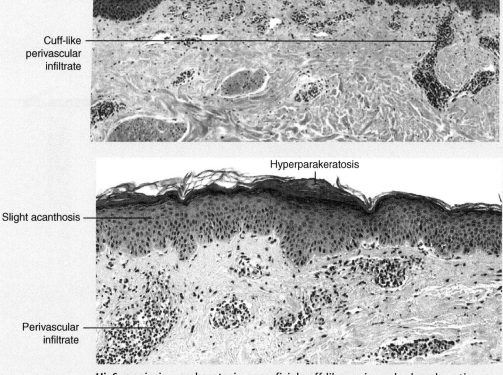

Hi: Spongiosis, parakeratosis, superficial cuff-like perivascular lymphocytic infiltrate; superficial and deep forms, cuff-like lymphocytic perivascular infiltrates in all dermal layers, no or subtle epidermal changes.

DIFFERENTIAL DIAGNOSIS: **Pityriasis lichenoides**

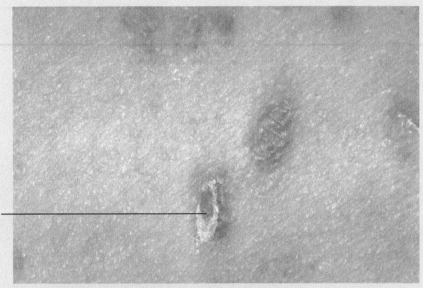

Tiny patches with scaling

Cl: Erythematous small patches or papules with scaling led and subsequent superficial ulceration. Spectrum of diseases includes acute (PLEVA, *see* chapter Necrotic, page 84), subacute and chronic forms.

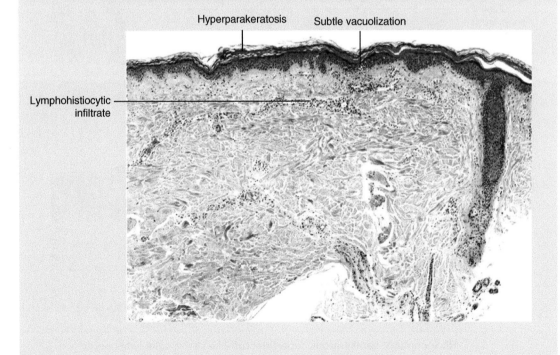

Hyperparakeratosis   Subtle vacuolization

Lymphohistiocytic infiltrate

Pityriasis lichenoides

Focal vacuolization

Predominantly
lymphocytic
infiltrate

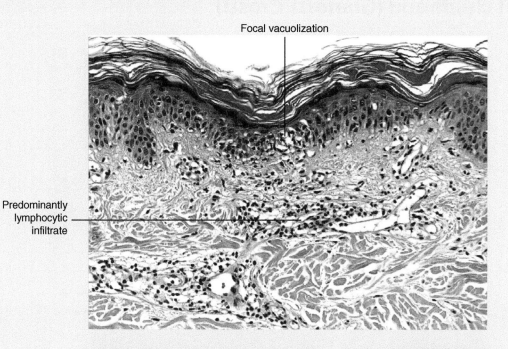

Vacuolization at
junctional zone

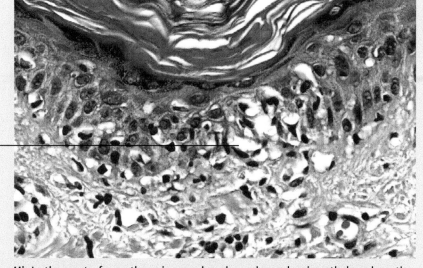

Hi: In the acute form, there is a wedge-shaped, predominantly lymphocytic
infiltrate, often band-like at the junction, focal hyperparakeratosis with
inclusions of neutrophils, intraepidermal erythrocyte extravasation, focal
vacuolization of the dermal–epidermal junction, exocytosis of lymphocytes
and single apoptotic keratinocytes. In chronic forms the changes are
more subtle, albeit with a subepidermal infiltrate.

DIFFERENTIAL DIAGNOSIS: Papular acrodermatitis of childhood (Gianotti-Crosti)

Small papules

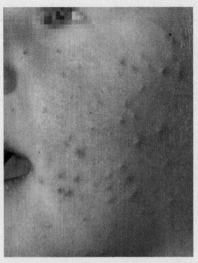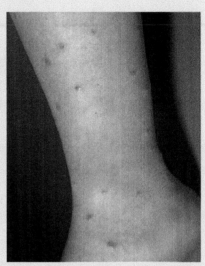

Cl: Small red papules in the face or on the limbs, fever, systemic involvement possible (hepatitis).

Focal epidermal necrosis

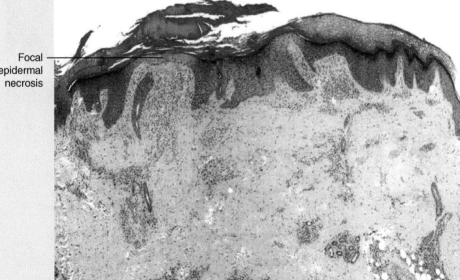

Hi: Early lesions: spongiosis, foci of epidermal necrosis, exocytosis of neutrophils and eosinophils as well as intraepidermal accumulations of Langerhans cells.

Other Diagnosis

Tinea: *Neutrophils in the horny layer, plasma cells, detection of fungi by PAS- or Grocott stain.*

References

Bonamonte, D., C. Foti, M. Vestita, *et al.* (2012). "Nummular eczema and contact allergy: a retrospective study." *Dermatitis* **23**(4): 153–7.

Clarke, L. E., K. F. Helm, J. Hennessy, *et al.* (2012). "Dermal dendritic cells in psoriasis, nummular dermatitis, and normal-appearing skin." *J Am Acad Dermatol* **66**(1): 98–105.

Jarvikallio, A., I. T. Harvima, and A. Naukkannen (2003). "Mast cells, nerves and neuropeptides in atopic dermatitis and nummular eczema." *Arch Dermatol Res* **295**(1): 2–7.

Maddison, B., A. Parsons, O. Sangueza, *et al.* (2011). "Retrospective study of intraepidermal nerve fiber distribution in biopsies of patients with nummular eczema." *Am J Dermatopathol* **33**(6): 621–3.

Patel, N., A. Mohammadi, and R. Rhatigan (2012). "A comparative analysis of mast cell quantification in five common dermatoses: lichen simplex chronicus, psoriasis, lichen planus, lupus, and insect bite/allergic contact dermatitis/nummular dermatitis." *ISRN Dermatol* **2012**: 759630.

Stevens, D. M. and A. B. Ackerman (1984). "On the concept of distinctive exudative discoid and lichenoid chronic dermatosis (Sulzberger-Garbe). Is it nummular dermatitis?" *Am J Dermatopathol* **6**(4): 387–95.

EPIDERMIS

PROTOTYPE: Eczema, chronic: Atopic dermatitis, Lichen simplex chronicus

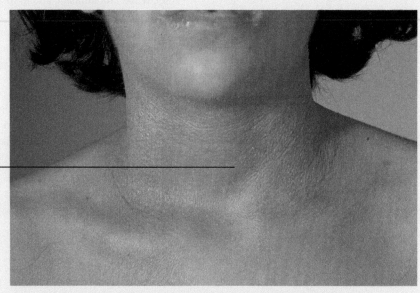

Hyperpigmented chronically inflamed skin; lichenification

CI: Pruritus, chronic well demarcated plaques, showing lichenification (thickening of skin, prominent skin lines) and hyperpigmentation (variable). Excoriations from scratching.

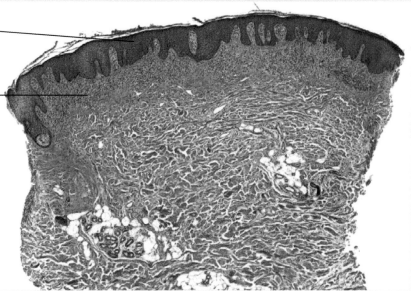

Psoriasiform and broad acanthosis and papillomatosis

Predominantly lymphocytic inflammatory infiltrate

Atopic dermatitis

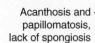
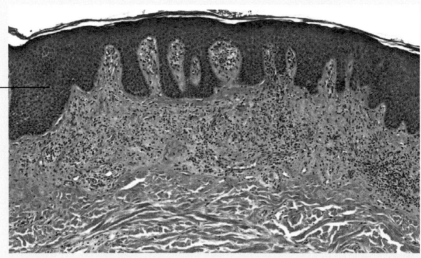

Acanthosis and
papillomatosis,
lack of spongiosis

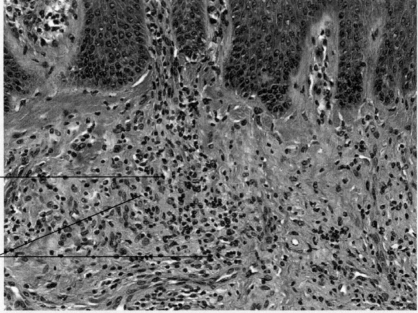

Predominantly
lymphocytic
inflammatory
infiltrate

Scattered
eosinophils

Hi: Acanthosis, hyperparakeratosis, no inclusions of serum, hypergranulosis, reduced or absence of spongiosis, mild perivascular infiltrate of lymphocytes, fibrosis of the papillary dermis. Scattered eosinophils may be present.

VARIANT: Subacute eczema

Focal and subtle spongiosis.

DIFFERENTIAL DIAGNOSIS: Cutaneous T-cell lymphoma (CTCL)

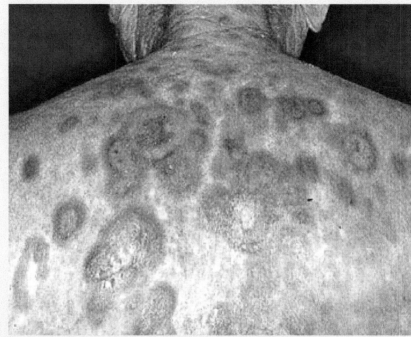

Circumscribed
flat infiltrates
(plaques)

Cl: Circumscribed patches and plaques with tendency to tumorous transformation.

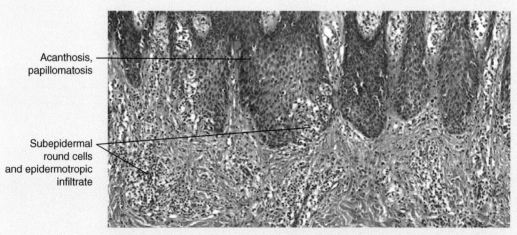

Acanthosis,
papillomatosis

Subepidermal
round cells
and epidermotropic
infiltrate

Hi: Nuclear atypia of lymphocytes which show lining-up at the junctional zone and formation of Pautrier microabscesses.

Other Diagnosis

Psoriasis (see Psoriasiform*): Inclusions of neutrophils in hyperparakeratosis, reduced or absent granular layer.*

Prurigo: Dermal fibrosis (see Pruriginous, page 42*).*

Parapsoriasis / chronic superficial dermatitis (see Psoriasiform, page 54*): Focal parakeratosis and exocytosis of lymphocytes, lack of significant acanthosis or spongiosis, sparse lymphocytic dermal infiltrate.*

Pityriasis rubra pilaris (see Psoriasiform, page 56*): Alternating ortho- and hyperparakeratosis (checkerboard sign), follicular plugging, plump rete ridges, sparse lymphocytic infiltrate.*

References

Hurwitz, R. M. and C. DeTrana (1990). "The cutaneous pathology of atopic dermatitis." *Am J Dermatopathol* **12**(6): 544–51.

Summey, B. T., S. E. Bowen, and H. B. Allen (2008). "Lichen planus-like atopic dermatitis: expanding the differential diagnosis of spongiotic dermatitis." *J Cutan Pathol* **35**(3): 311–14.

PROTOTYPE: Prurigo simplex subacuta/chronica

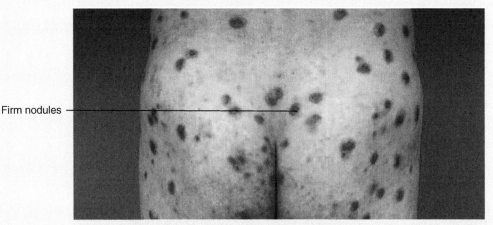

Firm nodules

Cl: Pruritic papules and nodules, red or hyperpigmented, preferentially on the trunk and extremities. Female>male preponderance.

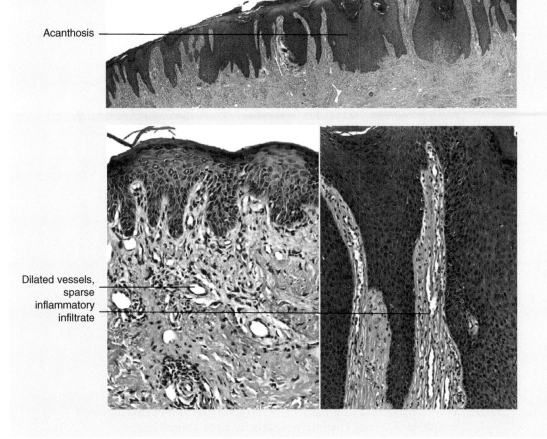

Acanthosis

Dilated vessels, sparse inflammatory infiltrate

EPIDERMIS

Prurigo simplex

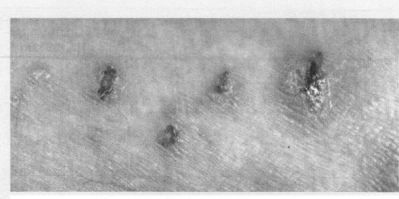

Excoriated
nodules

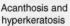

Acanthosis and
hyperkeratosis

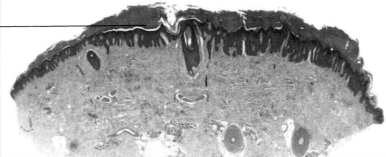

Plump and
hypertrophic
rete ridges

Dilated vessels

Fibrosis

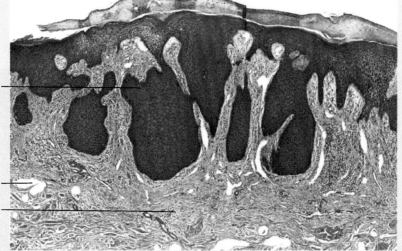

Hi: Pseudocarcinomatous acanthosis, focal hyperparakeratosis, hypergranulosis, papillomatosis, vertical papillary fibrosis, increased number of fibroblasts and subtle fibrosis, sparse lymphocytic infiltrate. A few eosinophils, plasma cells and ulceration may be present.

Comment

Additional examinations (history, serology) are recommended to search for diabetes mellitus, chronic hepatopathy and nephropathy.

VARIANT: **Prurigo nodularis, Hyde-type**

Clinical variant showing large nodules.

DIFFERENTIAL DIAGNOSIS: Infestation and arthropod bite reaction

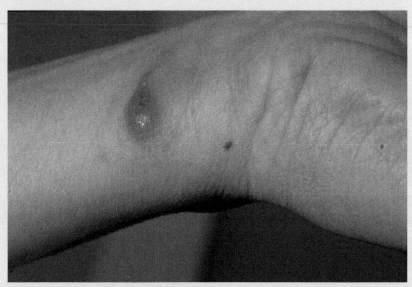

Late arthropod bite reaction: fibrotic nodule (histiocytoma)

Cl: Firm red nodule, occasionally excoriated.

Arthropod bite, early reaction

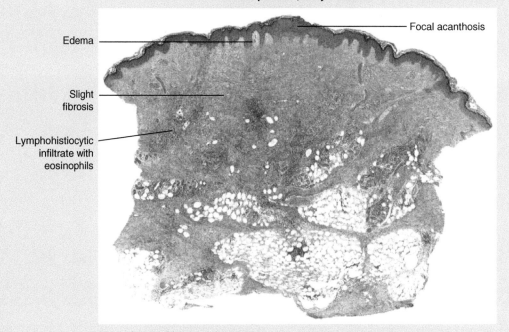

Focal acanthosis

Edema

Slight fibrosis

Lymphohistiocytic infiltrate with eosinophils

Hi: Arthropod bite, early reaction.

Infestation and arthropod bite reaction

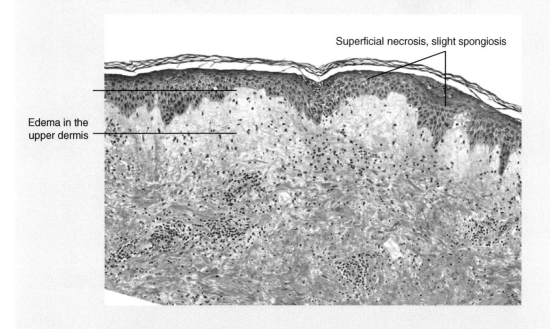

Superficial necrosis, slight spongiosis

Edema in the upper dermis

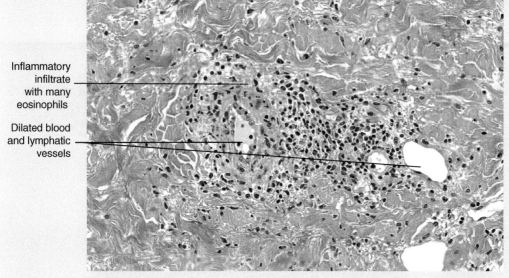

Inflammatory infiltrate with many eosinophils

Dilated blood and lymphatic vessels

Hi: Focal spongiosis or excoriation, mixed cellular infiltrate (early lesions) with numerous eosinophils. Fibrotic nodule (histiocytoma) is a late stage reaction.

EPIDERMIS

EPIDERMIS

DIFFERENTIAL DIAGNOSIS: Clavus/knuckle pads

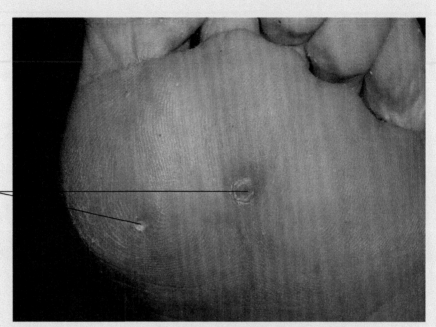

Endophytic
hard corns

Cl: Circumscribed brownish nodule or hyperkeratotic lesion on the plantar surface (clavus).

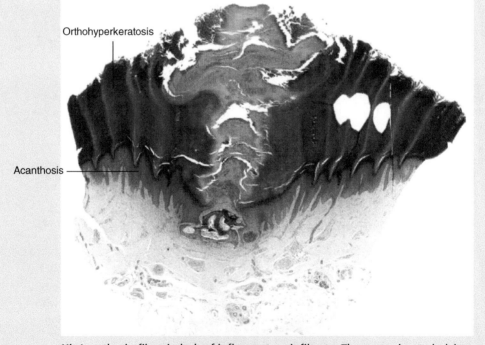

Orthohyperkeratosis

Acanthosis

Hi: Acanthosis, fibrosis, lack of inflammatory infiltrate. There may be underlying osteoma cutis in some cases.

DIFFERENTIAL DIAGNOSIS: **Epidermal nevus**

Verrucous lesions

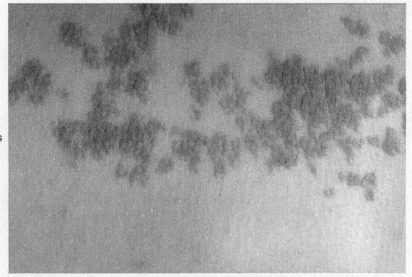

Cl: Brownish hyperkeratosis, sometimes linear or along tension lines.

Hyperkeratosis,
acanthosis
and papillomatosis

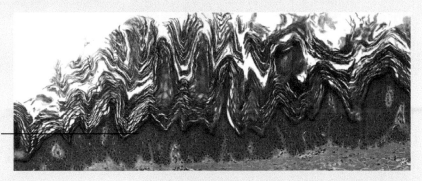

Epidermolytic
keratinocytes
(epidermolytic
epidermal nevus)

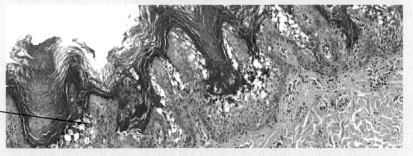

Hi: Circumscibed lesion, orthohyperkeratosis, lack of inflammatory infiltrate.

DIFFERENTIAL DIAGNOSIS: White sponge nevus of the mucous membrane

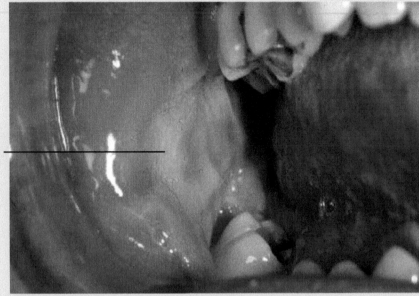

Whitish netlike area of mucous membrane of the cheek

Cl: White netlike spot on the mucous membrane.

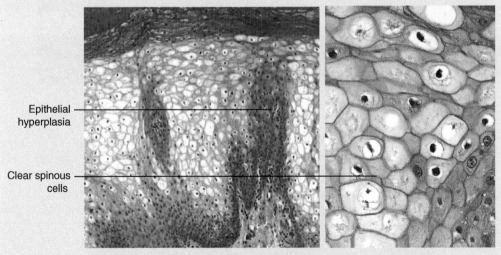

Epithelial hyperplasia

Clear spinous cells

Hi: Epithelial hyperplasia with clear spinous cells, showing perinuclear eosinophilic condensations.

Other Diagnosis

Reactive leukoplakia: Vacuolated and ballooned epithelial cells in the upper third of the epithelium, focal para- and/or hyperkeratosis, acanthosis.

Chronic eczema (see Chronic, page 36*)*

References

Lindley, R. P. and C. M. Payne (1989). "Neural hyperplasia is not a diagnostic prerequisite in nodular prurigo. A controlled morphometric microscopic study of 26 biopsy specimens." *J Cutan Pathol* **16**(1): 14–18.

Weigelt, N., D. Metze, and S. Ständer (2010). "Prurigo nodularis: systematic analysis of 58 histological criteria in 136 patients." *J Cutan Pathol* **37**(5): 578–86.

PROTOTYPE: **Psoriasis vulgaris**

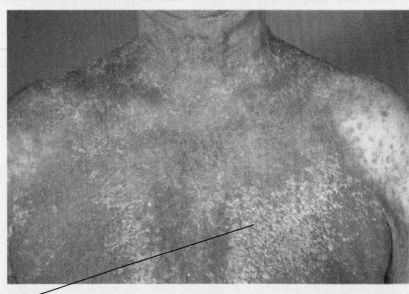

Erythemato-
squamous plaques
and papules

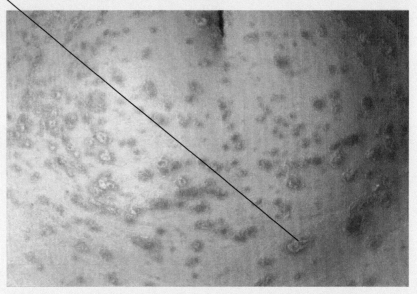

Cl: Sharply demarcated scaling and erythematous papules and plaques.

Psoriasis vulgaris

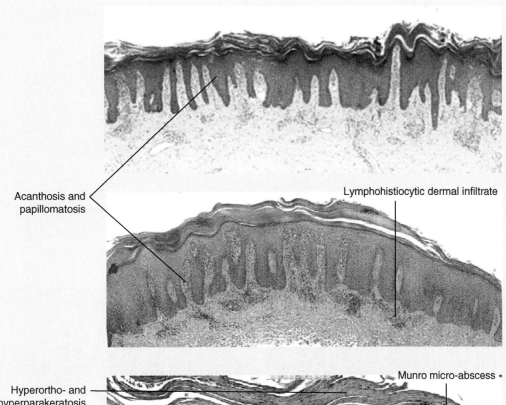

Acanthosis and papillomatosis

Lymphohistiocytic dermal infiltrate

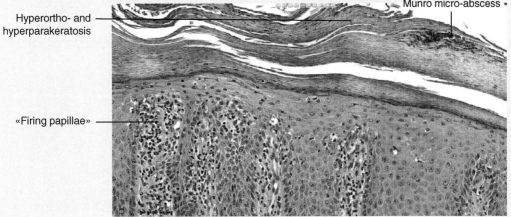

Hyperortho- and hyperparakeratosis

Munro micro-abscess

«Firing papillae»

Psoriasis vulgaris

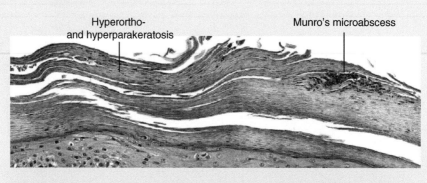

Hyperortho-
and hyperparakeratosis

Munro's microabscess

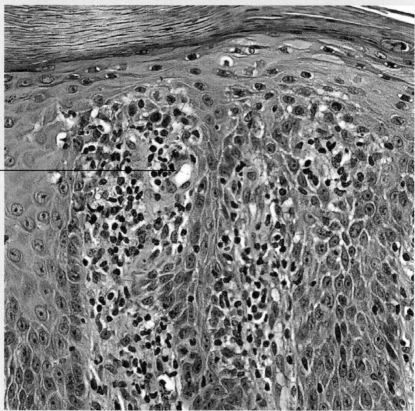

Dilated capillary

Psoriasis vulgaris

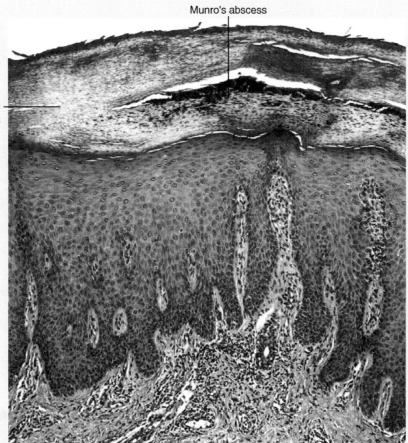

Munro's abscess

Hyperortho- and
hyperparakeratosis

Hi: Hyperortho- and hyperparakeratosis. Acanthosis and papillomatosis.
Neutrophilic micro-abscesses in the cornified layer (Munro's micro-abscesses)
and in the upper spinous layer (Kogoj's pustules). Focal loss of stratum
granulosum. Tortuous elongation and dilatation of papillary capillaries.
Thinning of the epidermis above tips of the papillae. Lymphocytic infiltrate in
the papillary dermis ("firering" (Grüneberg) or "squirting" (Pinkus) papillae).

VARIANTS

Psoriasis pustulosa generalisata (von Zumbusch) (see Pustular, page 70)
Psoriasis pustulosa palmo-plantaris (Königsbeck-Barber) (see Pustular, page 70)

DIFFERENTIAL DIAGNOSIS: Parapsoriasis, large plaque (mycosis fungoides early stage)

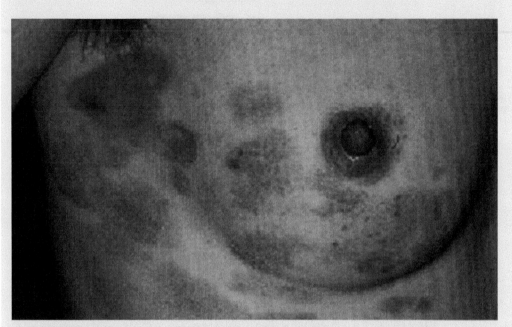

Cl: Confluent, erythematous patches, sometimes slightly scaling.

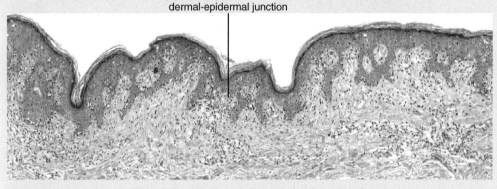

Epidermotropic infiltrate at the dermal-epidermal junction

Hi: Epidermis normal or slightly acanthotic, superficial lymphocytic infiltrate with epidermotropism, preferentially along on the tip of the rete ridges. Edema and slight fibrosis may be present in the papillary dermis.

Comment

Psoriasis and parapsoriasis (PP) are semantic differential diagnoses. Large plaque parapsoriasis is widely considered as early stage of mycosis fungoides and clinically may simulate psoriasis; histologically, however, PP presents completely differently from psoriasis (see Lichenoid, page 120).

DIFFERENTIAL DIAGNOSIS: **Seborrheic dermatitis, subacute dermatitis**

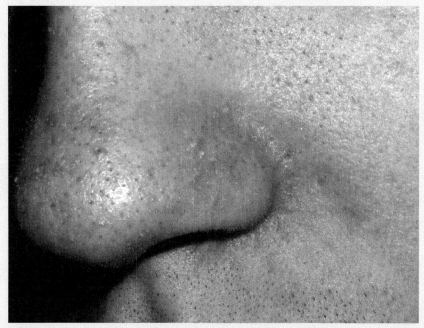

Erythema, slightly scaling

Cl: Erythema and scaling, preferentially in central face and scalp.

Hyperparakeratosis, scaling

Psoriasiform acanthosis and papillomatosis

Hi: Acanthosis, papillomatosis and parahyperkeratosis, particularly around hair follicle ostia, exocytosis of neutrophils.

EPIDERMIS

DIFFERENTIAL DIAGNOSIS: Pityriasis rubra pilaris

Erythematous patches

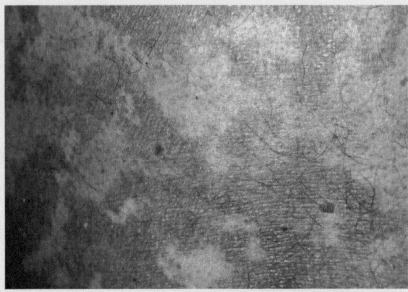

CI: Psoriasiform erythema, follicularly bound with uninvolved skin in between (nappes claires).

Acanthosis and papillomatosis

Horizontally and vertically alternating ortho- and hyper-parakeratosis

Sparse inflammatory infiltrate

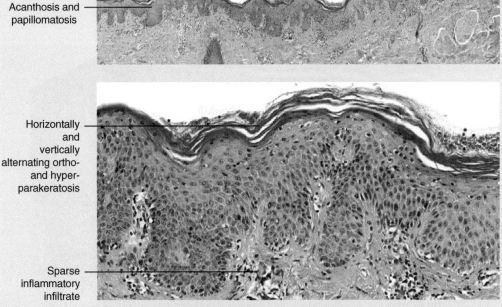

Hi: Plump acanthosis and papillomatosis, horizontally and vertically alternating ortho- and hyperparakeratosis (checkerboard sign), no or rather sparse lymphocytic infiltrate.

Other Diagnosis

Nummular dermatitis: Spongiosis, hyperparakeratosis *(see* Subacute, page 25*)*.

Chronic atopic dermatitis; lichen simplex chronicus (see Chronic, page 36*): No inclusion of neutrophils, broadened granular layer, broad acanthosis.*

Fungus infection: Little inflammation, demonstration of hyphae and spores in the stratum corneum by PAS-stain *(see* Pustular, page 75*)*.

Epidermal nevus: Verruciform profile, lack of inflammation, sometimes epidermolytic changes of keratinocytes *(see* Koilocytic, page 102*)*.

Reiter's syndrome: Involvement of genital and oral mucosa. Histology identical to psoriasis.

References

Braun-Falco, O. and G. Burg (1970). "[Histochemistry of capillaries in psoriasis vulgaris]." *Arch Klin Exp Dermatol* **236**(2): 173–89.

Braun-Falco, O. and G. Burg (1970). "[Inflammatory infiltrate in psoriasis vulgaris. A cytochemical study]." *Arch Klin Exp Dermatol* **236**(3): 297–314.

Kouskoukis, C. E., R. K. Scher, and A. B. Ackerman (1983). "What histologic finding distinguishes onychomycosis and psoriasis?" *Am J Dermatopathol* **5**(5): 501–3.

Magro, C. M. and A. N. Crowson (1997). "The clinical and histomorphological features of pityriasis rubra pilaris. A comparative analysis with psoriasis." *J Cutan Pathol* **24**(7): 416–24.

Mordovtsev, V. N. and V. I. Albanova (1989). "Morphology of skin microvasculature in psoriasis." *Am J Dermatopathol* **11**(1): 33–42.

Pinkus, H. and A. H. Mehregan (1980). "On the evolution, maturation, and regression of lesions of psoriasis." *Am J Dermatopathol* **2**(3): 287–8.

Ragaz, A. and A. B. Ackerman (1979). "Evolution, maturation, and regression of lesions of psoriasis. New observations and correlation of clinical and histologic findings." *Am J Dermatopathol* **1**(3): 199–214.

Sweet, W. L. and B. R. Smoller (1997). "Differential proliferation of endothelial cells and keratinocytes in psoriasis and spongiotic dermatitis." *J Cutan Pathol* **24**(6): 356–63.

EPIDERMIS

PROTOTYPE: **Pemphigus vulgaris**

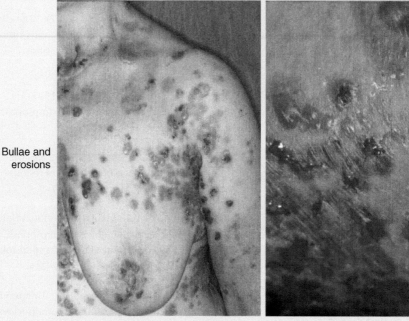

Bullae and erosions

Cl: Onset with oral erosions in 50% of cases, later superficial, fragile blisters with rapid transition to crusted erosions.

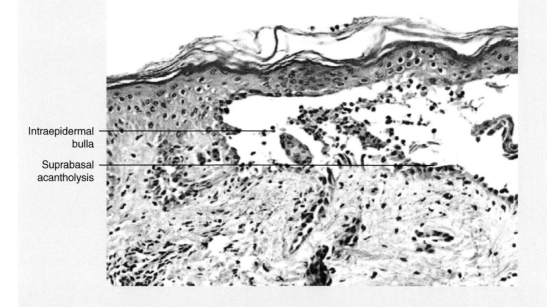

Intraepidermal bulla

Suprabasal acantholysis

Pemphigus vulgaris

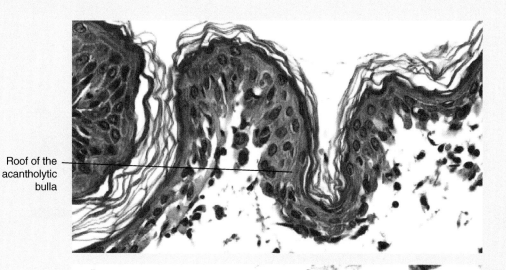

Roof of the acantholytic bulla

Bottom of the acantholytic bulla

Intercellular deposits of antibodies

Acantholytic cells

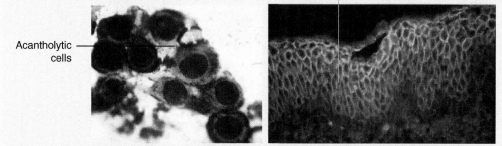

Hi: Intraepidermal suprabasal clefts due to acantholysis. Acantholytic cells floating in the blisters. Tombstone-like arrangement of basal keratinocytes. Labelling of IgG autoantibodies against surface proteins of keratinocytes in the direct immunofluorescence.

EPIDERMIS

VARIANT: **Pemphigus foliaceus**

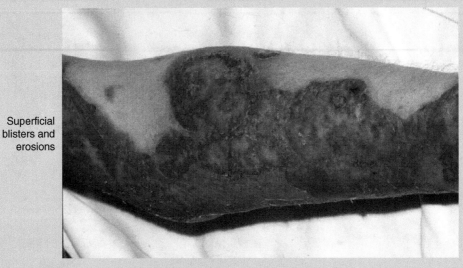

Superficial blisters and erosions

Cl: Superficial erosions and crusts.

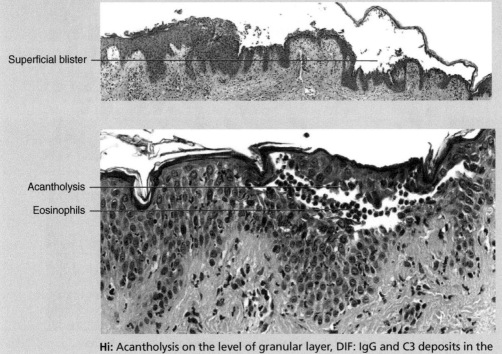

Superficial blister —

Acantholysis —
Eosinophils —

Hi: Acantholysis on the level of granular layer, DIF: IgG and C3 deposits in the upper layers of the epidermis.

VARIANT: **Pemphigus vegetans**

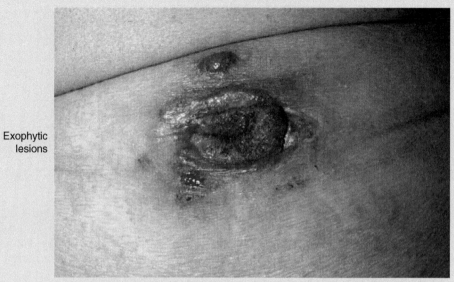

Exophytic
lesions

Cl: Vesicles, blisters or pustules with papillomatous growth and vegetations.

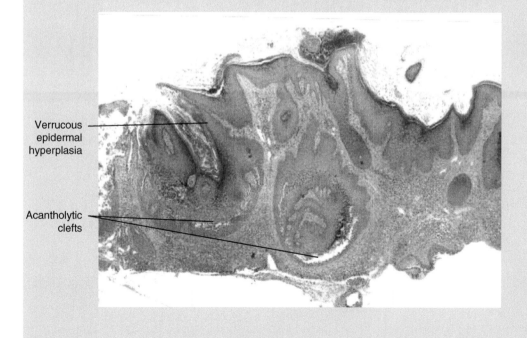

Verrucous
epidermal
hyperplasia

Acantholytic
clefts

Pemphigus vegetans

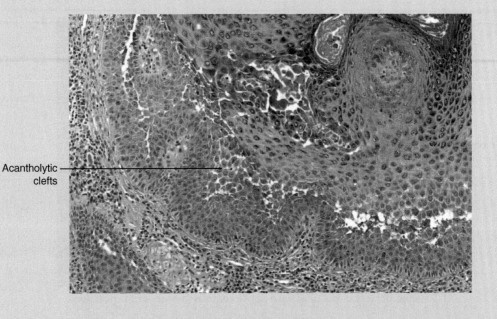

Acantholytic clefts

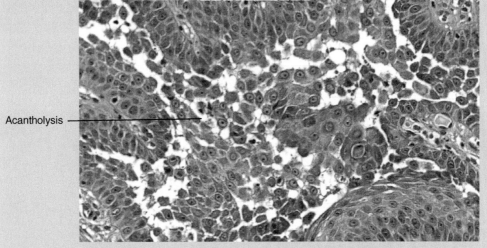

Acantholysis

Hi: Suprabasal acantholytic blisters, verrucous epidermal hyperplasia, pustules with eosinophils.

VARIANT: **IgA Pemphigus**

IgA Pemphigus

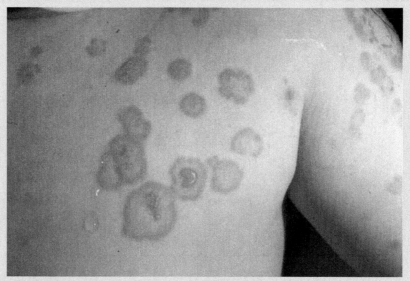

Cl: Vesicles or pustules, annular arrangement.

Superficial
acantholytic
blister

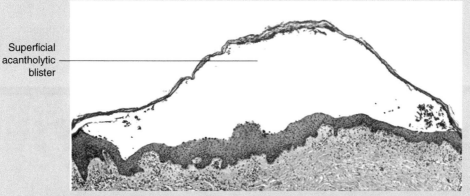

Hi: Subepidermal acantholytic blister. DIF: IgA deposits in the upper layers of the epidermis.

Paraneoplastic pemphigus: *Suprabasal acantholysis, interface dermatitis.*

EPIDERMIS

DIFFERENTIAL DIAGNOSIS: Chronic benign familial pemphigus (Hailey-Hailey's disease)

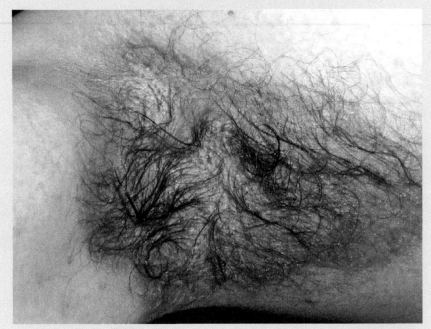

Oozing erythema in the axilla

Cl: Maceration and friction, preferentially in the groin, axilla, perianal region, and the neck.

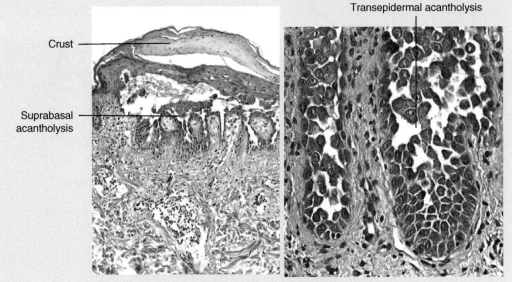

Crust

Suprabasal acantholysis

Transepidermal acantholysis

Hi: Suprabasal acantholysis, dyskeratosis, hyperparakeratosis.

DIFFERENTIAL DIAGNOSIS: Dyskeratosis follicularis (Darier's disease)

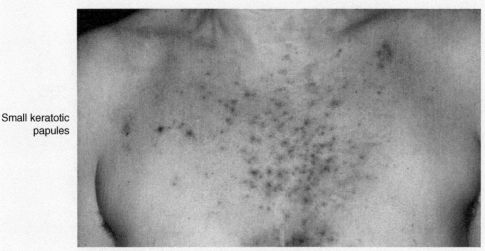

Small keratotic papules

Cl: Grayish tiny keratotic papules preferentially in the seborrheic (central axis) areas of the breast and back.

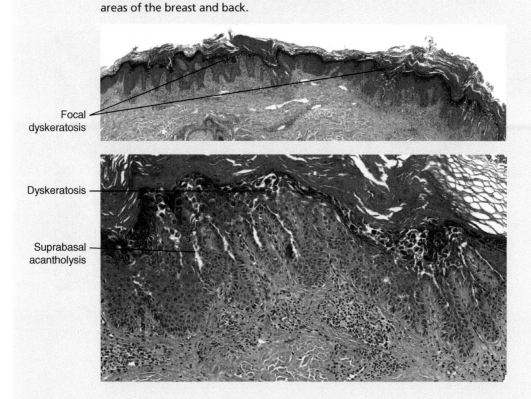

Focal dyskeratosis

Dyskeratosis

Suprabasal acantholysis

Dyskeratosis follicularis

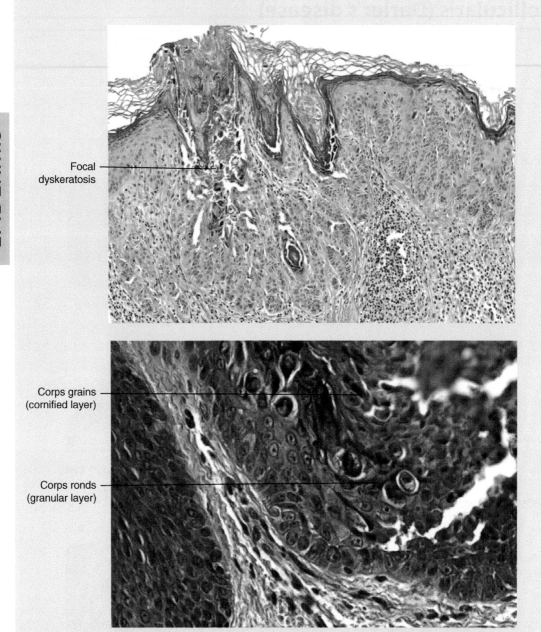

Focal dyskeratosis

Corps grains (cornified layer)

Corps ronds (granular layer)

Hi: Acantholytic dyskeratosis, suprabasal cleft, acanthosis, parakeratosis, corps ronds and grains due to dyskeratosis.

DIFFERENTIAL DIAGNOSIS: **Transient acantholytic dermatosis (Grover's disease)**

Tiny papules
on the chest

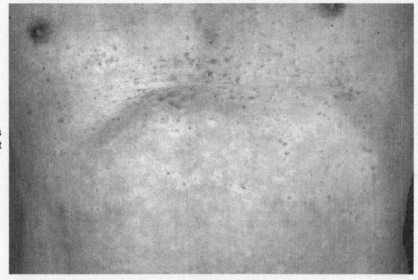

CI: Multiple tiny pruritic papules or vesicles on the trunk.

Small focus
of suprabasal
acantholysis
and dyskeratosis

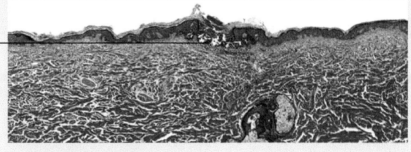

Suprabasal
acantholysis,
dyskeratosis,
funnel-like
hyperparakeratosis

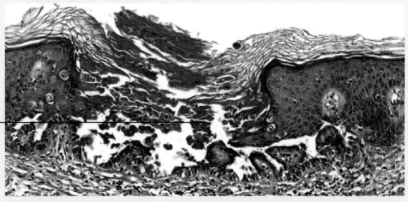

Hi: Small acantholytic foci with dyskeratosis, seen also in Darier's or Hailey-Hailey's disease.

Other Diagnosis

Bullous pemphigoid: *Subepidermal blister without acantholysis; eosinophils and neutrophils in the blister cavity and in the dermal infiltrate, no necrotic keratinocytes, no significant edema in the dermis, admixture of plasma cells.*

Impetigo contagiosa *(see Pustular, page 73): Subcorneal acantholysis, neutrophils and exsudate in the superficial blister, mixed dermal infiltrate with neutrophils, eosinophils and plasma cells. Bacteria may be detected in the blister.*

Other bullous skin diseases

References

Kouskoukis, C. E. and A. B. Ackerman (1984). "What histologic finding distinguishes superficial pemphigus and bullous impetigo?" *Am J Dermatopathol* **6**(2): 179–81.

Landau, M. and S. Brenner (1997). "Histopathologic findings in drug-induced pemphigus." *Am J Dermatopathol* **19**(4): 411–14.

Lanza, A., N. Cirillo, F. Memiano, and F. Gombos (2006). "How does acantholysis occur in pemphigus vulgaris: a critical review." *J Cutan Pathol* **33**(6): 401–12.

Mahalingam, M. (2005). "Follicular acantholysis: a subtle clue to the early diagnosis of pemphigus vulgaris." *Am J Dermatopathol* **27**(3): 237–9.

Montes, L. F. (1976). "Familial benign chronic pemphigus (Hailey-Hailey disease)." *J Cutan Pathol* **3**(2): 116–17.

Rubinstein, N. and J. R. Stanley (1987). "Pemphigus foliaceus antibodies and a monoclonal antibody to desmoglein I demonstrate stratified squamous epithelial-specific epitopes of desmosomes." *Am J Dermatopathol* **9**(6): 510–14.

Smolle, J. and H. Kerl (1984). "Pitfalls in the diagnosis of pemphigus vulgaris (early pemphigus vulgaris with features of bullous pemphigoid)." *Am J Dermatopathol* **6**(5): 429–35.

PROTOTYPE: **Psoriasis pustulosa**

EPIDERMIS

VARIANT: Pustular psoriasis of palms and soles, Königsbeck-Barber-type

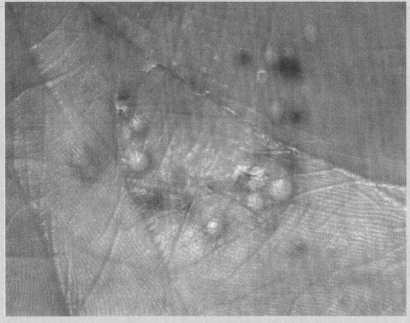

Pustules on palms and soles

Cl: Pustules on palms and soles (Königsbeck-Barber type) or generalized (von Zumbusch type).

Ruptured pustule with cellular debris

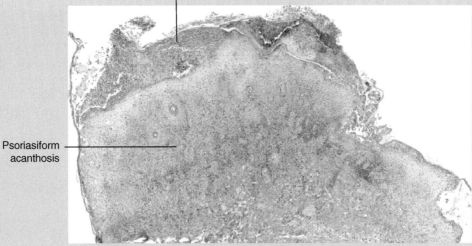

Psoriasiform acanthosis

Hi: Intraepidermal neutrophilic pustules (Kogoj pustules and Munro's micro-abscesses), psoriasiform acanthosis, hyperparakeratosis, perivascular lymphohistiocytic infiltrate with a few neutrophils in the upper dermis.

VARIANT: Generalized pustular psoriasis, von Zumbusch-type

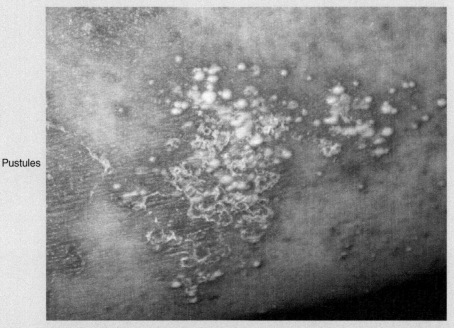

Pustules

Cl: Clinical variant; generalized pustules.

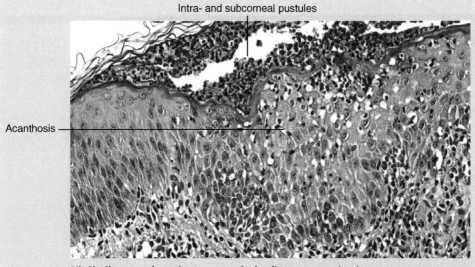

Intra- and subcorneal pustules

Acanthosis

Hi: Similar to palmoplantar pustulosis, discrete acanthosis.

EPIDERMIS

DIFFERENTIAL DIAGNOSIS: **Subcorneal pustulosis**

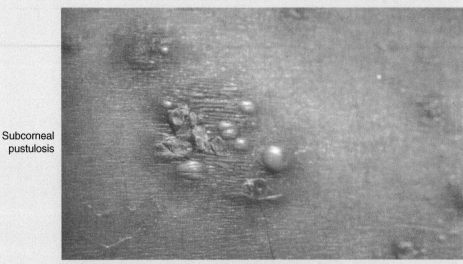

Subcorneal pustulosis

Cl: By some experts considered as a variant of pustular psoriasis.

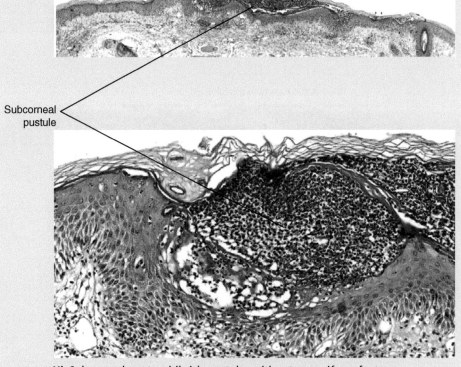

Subcorneal pustule

Hi: Subcorneal neutrophil-rich pustules without spongiform features.

Comment
IgA-pemphigus pattern.

DIFFERENTIAL DIAGNOSIS: **Impetigo contagiosa**

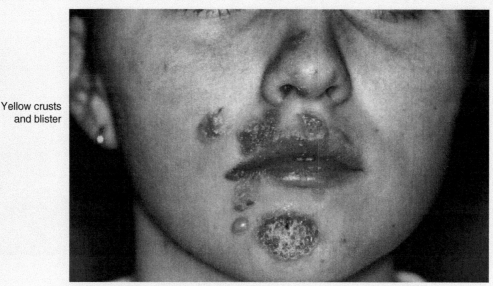

Yellow crusts and blister

Cl: Superficial erosion following destruction of small pustules, yellow circumscribed crusts.

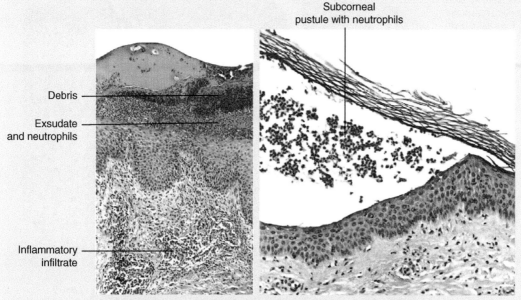

Subcorneal pustule with neutrophils

Debris

Exsudate and neutrophils

Inflammatory infiltrate

Hi: Subcorneal acantholysis, neutrophils and exsudate in the superficial blister, mixed dermal infiltrate with neutrophils, eosinophils and plasma cells. Bacteria may be detected in the blister.

EPIDERMIS

DIFFERENTIAL DIAGNOSIS: **Ostiofolliculitis (pustular)**

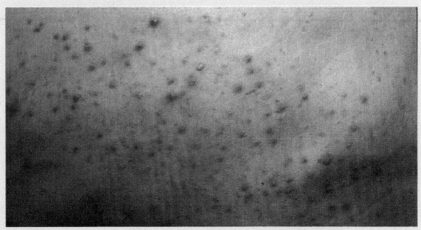

Tiny follicular papules and pustules

Cl: Follicle-bound small pustules.

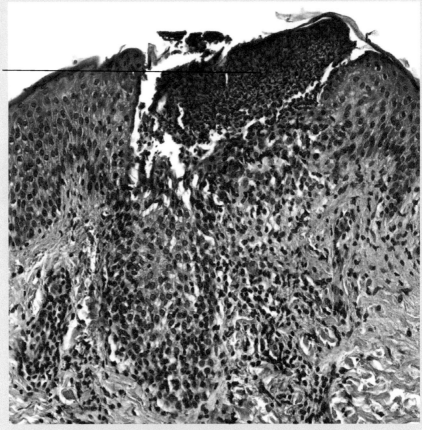

Inflammatory cells and debris in the follicular ostium

Hi: Involvement of follicular structures. Pustules in the follicular ostia.

DIFFERENTIAL DIAGNOSIS: **Tinea**

Superficial fungal infection with *dermatophytes*

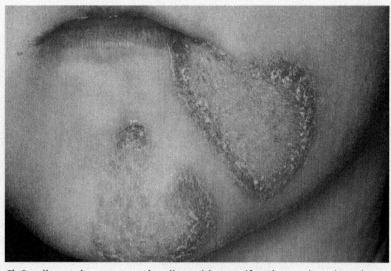

CI: Small pustules, crusts and scaling with centrifugal growth and tendency to regression in the center of the circumscribed lesions.

Superficial crust —

Sparse dermal infiltrate —

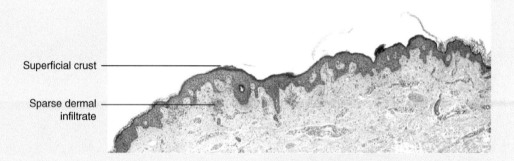

Hyphae in the cornified layer. *PAS-stain* —

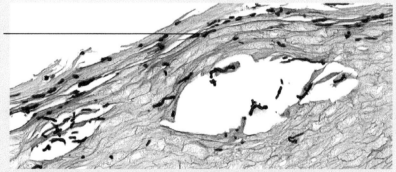

Hi: Focal crust formation, mixed cellular dermal infiltrate of neutrophils, occasionally eosinophils and plasma cells. Detection of fungi by PAS or Grocott stains.

DIFFERENTIAL DIAGNOSIS: Behçet's disease (Behçet-Adamantiades syndrome)

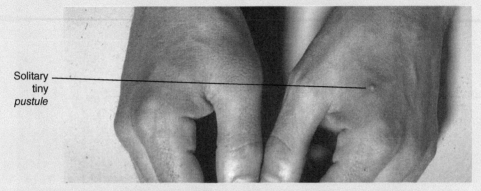

Solitary tiny *pustule*

Cl: Disseminated small pustules. Multisystemic disorder with oral and genital aphthae, uveitis, synovitis, thrombophlebitis and cutaneous pustular vasculitis in some cases.

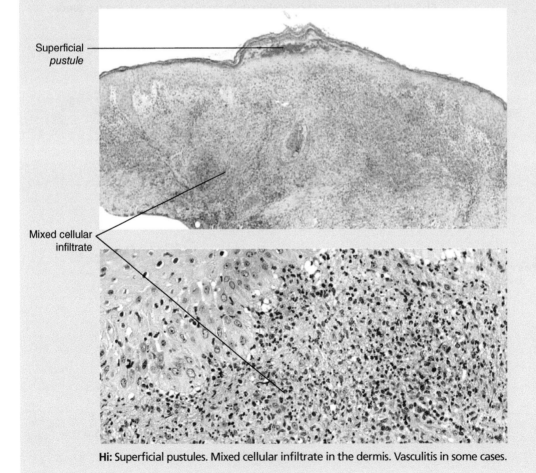

Superficial *pustule*

Mixed cellular infiltrate

Hi: Superficial pustules. Mixed cellular infiltrate in the dermis. Vasculitis in some cases.

Other Diagnosis

Acute generalized exanthematous pustulosis (AGEP): Often induced by drugs. Initially often starting in flexural body regions. Overlapping histology with pustular psorasis. Admixture of eosinophils. Discrete acanthosis.

Infantile acropustulosis: Early lesions: Spongiosis, foci of epidermal necrosis, exocytosis of neutrophils and eosinophils. Late lesions: subcorneal and intraepidermal pustules.

Transient neonatal pustular melanosis, early lesions: Distinct clinical features in a newborn.

Pemphigus foliaceus (see Bullous, acantholytic, page 60*): Acantholysis on the level of granular layer, DIF: IgG and C3 deposits in the upper layers of the epidermis.*

IgA Pemphigus: Acantholysis, subcorneal pustules with neutrophils. DIF: IgA deposits in the upper layers of the epidermis (see Bullous, page 63*).*

Miliaria cristallina and rubra (see Ekzematous, Acute, page 23*): Involvement of the acrosyringium, spongiosis, mixed cellular infiltrate with numerous neutrophils.*

References

Aydin, O., B. Engin, O. Oyuz, *et al.* (2008). "Non-pustular palmoplantar psoriasis: is histologic differentiation from eczematous dermatitis possible?" *J Cutan Pathol* **35**(2): 169–73.

Kardaun, S. H., H. Kuiper, V. Fidler, *et al.* (2010). "The histopathological spectrum of acute generalized exanthematous pustulosis (AGEP) and its differentiation from generalized pustular psoriasis." *J Cutan Pathol* **37**(12): 1220–9.

Kim, B. and P. E. LeBoit (2000). "Histopathologic features of erythema nodosum-like lesions in Behcet disease: A comparison with erythema nodosum focusing on the role of vasculitis." *Am J Dermatopathol* **22**(5): 379–90.

Leclerc-Mercier, S., C. Bodemer, E. Bourdon-Lanoy, *et al.* (2010). "Early skin biopsy is helpful for the diagnosis and management of neonatal and infantile erythrodermas." *J Cutan Pathol* **37**(2): 249–55.

Sanchez, N. P., H. O. Perry, S. A. Muller, *et al.* (1981). "On the relationship between subcorneal pustular dermatosis and pustular psoriasis." *Am J Dermatopathol* **3**(4): 385–6.

Sidoroff, A., S. Halevy, J. N. Bavinck, *et al.* (2001). "Acute generalized exanthematous pustulosis (AGEP) – a clinical reaction pattern." *J Cutan Pathol* **28**(3): 113–19.

Wolff, K. (1981). "Subcorneal pustular dermatosis is not pustular psoriasis." *Am J Dermatopathol* **3**(4): 381–2.

EPIDERMIS

PROTOTYPE: Toxic epidermal necrolysis (TEN, Lyell's syndrome)

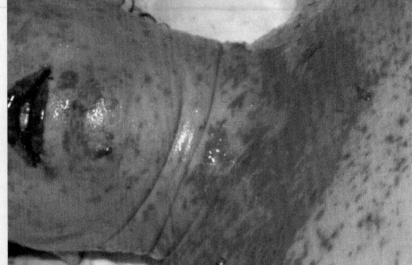

Widespread
superficial
necrosis

Cl: Starting with a confluent grayish, maculopapular exanthema, finally hemorrhagic blisters, epidermal necrosis and erosions due to loss of sheets of epidermis develop. Usually severe periorificial mucosal erosions.

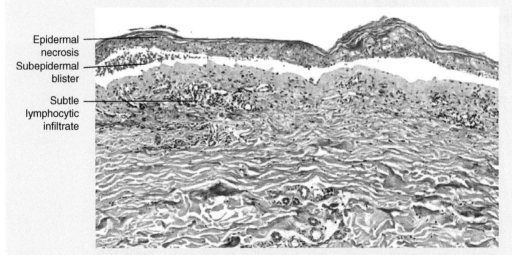

Epidermal
necrosis

Subepidermal
blister

Subtle
lymphocytic
infiltrate

Comment

Erythema exsudativum multiforme, Stevens-Johnson syndrome and toxic epidermal necrolysis are variants of the same disease spectrum but of varying severity.

Toxic epidermal necrolysis

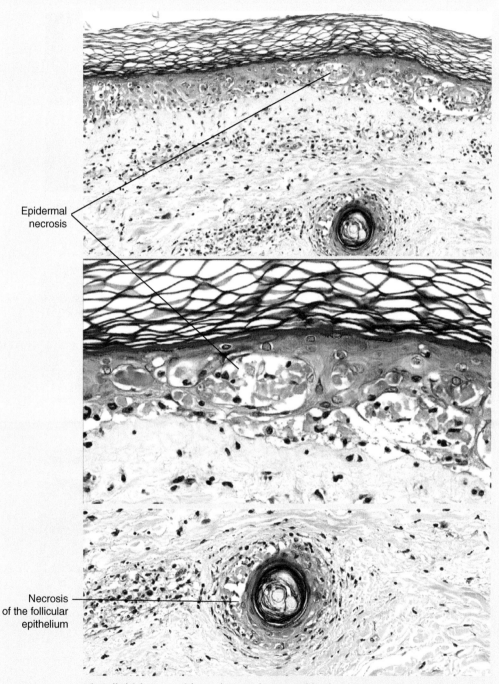

Epidermal
necrosis

Necrosis
of the follicular
epithelium

Hi: Full thickness epidermal necrosis, normal basket weave stratum corneum, subepidermal blister formation, dermal papillae intact, minimal inflammation, erythrocyte extravasation.

EPIDERMIS

VARIANT: **Erythema multiforme**

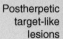

Postherpetic target-like lesions

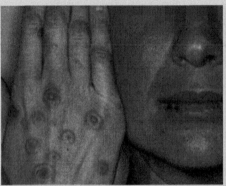
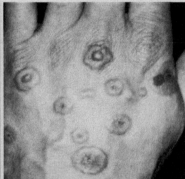

Cl: Erythematous blistering target- or iris-shaped lesions, preferentially on the dorsum of the hands.

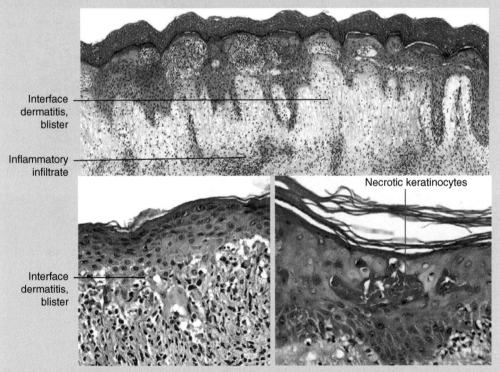

Interface dermatitis, blister

Inflammatory infiltrate

Necrotic keratinocytes

Interface dermatitis, blister

Hi: Interface dermatitis, necrotic keratinocytes in all epidermal layers, lymphocytic infiltrate, edema in the upper dermis.

VARIANT: Fixed drug reaction

Circumscribed
purpuric
brownish lesion

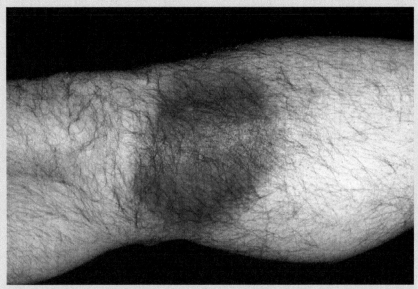

Cl: Solitary circumscribed often hemorrhagic erythema in a "fixed" localization.

Bullous interface
dermatitis

Inflammatory
infiltrate

Necrotic
keratinocytes

Eosinophils

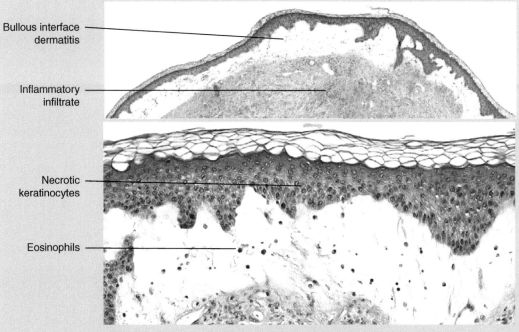

Hi: Single cell necrosis of keratinocytes in all epidermal layers, interface
dermatitis, lymphocytic infiltrate with eosinophils, pigment loss.

DIFFERENTIAL DIAGNOSIS

Staphylococcal scaled skin syndrome (SSSS): *Following a staphylococcal infection and mediated by bacterial exo-toxins, initially erythema resembling scarlet fever followed by unstable large blisters which quickly erode and lead to widespread loss of superficial parts of the epidermis.*
Histology shows subcorneal blistering with few granulocytes, few acantholytic keratinocytes, sparse perivascular infiltrate of neutrophils and lymphocytes.

DIFFERENTIAL DIAGNOSIS: (Phyto-) phototoxic dermatitis

Tense blisters

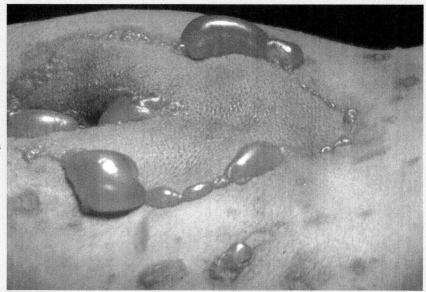

Cl: Erythema and tense blister formation in light exposed area, limited to the site contact of phototoxic agent (furocumarine) exposure.

Necrotic keratinocytes and epidermal necrosis

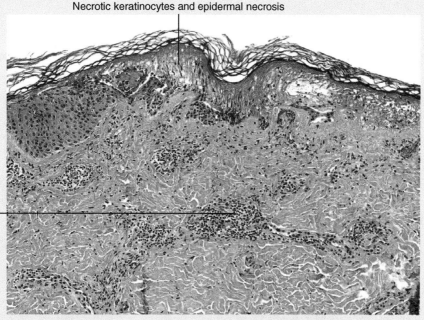

Inflammatory perivascular infiltrate

Hi: Necrotic keratinocytes, extensive edema or subepidermal blister formation, sparse infiltrate.

EPIDERMIS

DIFFERENTIAL DIAGNOSIS: **Pityriasis lichenoides et varioliformis acuta (PLEVA)**

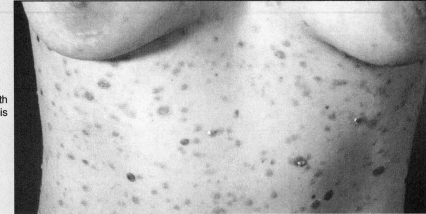

Papules with central necrosis

Cl: Small papules and plaques with scaling or superficial crust.

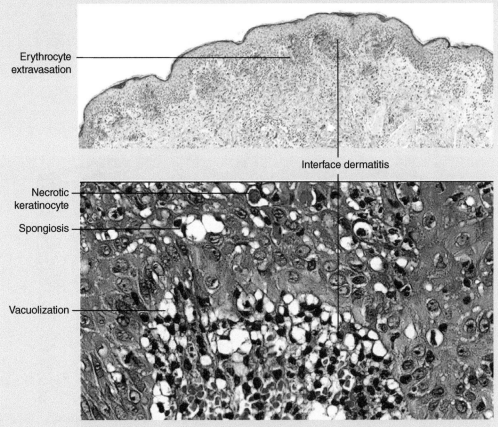

Erythrocyte extravasation

Interface dermatitis

Necrotic keratinocyte

Spongiosis

Vacuolization

Hi: Focal epidermal changes (vacuolization, spongiosis, exocytosis of lymphocytes), necrotic keratinocytes, focal hyperparakeratosis with inclusions of neutrophils, erythrocyte extravasation.

DIFFERENTIAL DIAGNOSIS: **Necrolytic migratory erythema (Glucagonoma-syndrome)**

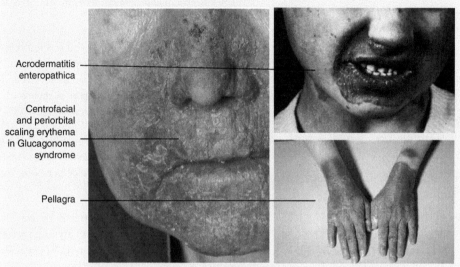

Acrodermatitis enteropathica

Centrofacial and periorbital scaling erythema in Glucagonoma syndrome

Pellagra

Cl: Eczematous changes periorally and around other orifices.

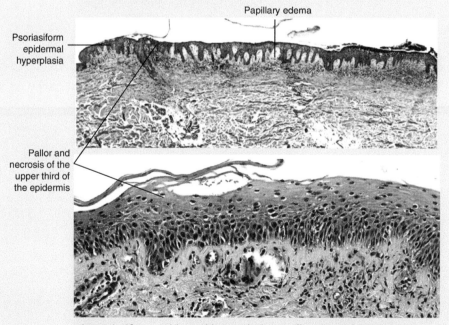

Papillary edema

Psoriasiform epidermal hyperplasia

Pallor and necrosis of the upper third of the epidermis

Hi: Psoriasiform epidermal hyperplasia, confluent parakeratosis, pallor and/or necrosis of the upper third of the epidermis, superficial perivascular infiltrate, papillary edema.

Comment
Superficial necrobiosis of the epidermis with crust formation is the common denominator of these etiologically different disorders.

Other Diagnosis

Acrodermatitis enteropathica (zinc deficiency-syndrome): Histologic changes similar to necrolytic migratory erythema.

Pellagra: Histologic changes similar to necrolytic migratory erythema.

Viral exanthema, herpes virus: Acantholysis, ballooning of keratinocytes, multinucleated syncytial epithelial cells, homogenized steel-grey nucleoplasm, marginalized chromatin (see Ballooning, page 87).

Graft-versus-host reaction, acute: Interface dermatitis, necrotic keratinocytes. Clinical context (see Chapter Lichenoid, page 116).

Combustio and congelatio: Epidermal necrosis. History, clinical context.

Porphyria cutanea tarda (see Chapter 3, Subepidermal blistering, page 128).

References

Letko, E., D. N. Papaliodis, G. N. Papaliodism, *et al.* (2005). "Stevens-Johnson syndrome and toxic epidermal necrolysis: a review of the literature." *Ann Allergy Asthma Immunol* **94**(4): 419–36; quiz 436–438, 456.

Lyell, A. (1983). "The staphylococcal scalded skin syndrome in historical perspective: emergence of dermopathic strains of Staphylococcus aureus and discovery of the epidermolytic toxin. A review of events up to 1970." *J Am Acad Dermatol* **9**(2): 285–94.

Megahed, M. (2004). *Histopathology of Blistering Diseases: With Clinical, Electron Microscopic, Immunological and Molecular Biological Correlations.* Heidelber, New York, Springer.

Papadopoulos, A. J., R. A. Schwartz, Z. Fekete, *et al.* (2001). "Pseudoporphyria: an atypical variant resembling toxic epidermal necrolysis." *J Cutan Med Surg* **5**(6): 479–85.

PROTOTYPE: **Alpha-herpes virus-infections: Herpes simplex**

Groups of blisters on erythema

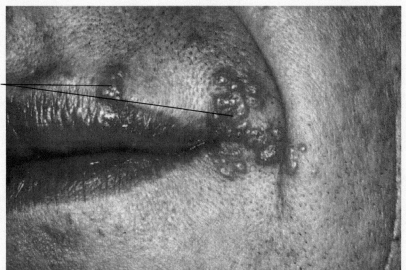

Cl: Erythema with clusters of small vesicles, usually on the lips (type 1) or the genital mucosa (type 2).

Intraepidermal blisters

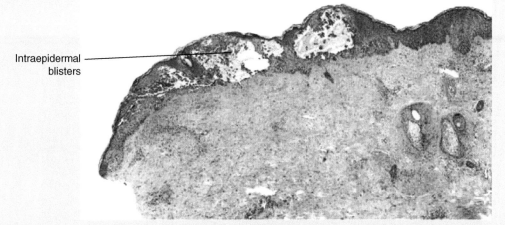

Hi: Acantholysis, ballooning degeneration of keratinocytes, "steel gray" nuclei of keratinocytes, necrotic keratinocytes, multinucleated (syncytial) epithelial cells, inter- and intracellular edema and intraepidermal vesicles. Mixed cellular infiltrate, lymphocytes predominating, dermal edema, occasionally lymphocytic and leukocytoklastic vasculitis.

EPIDERMIS

VARIANTS: Varicella (Chickenpox)/Herpes zoster

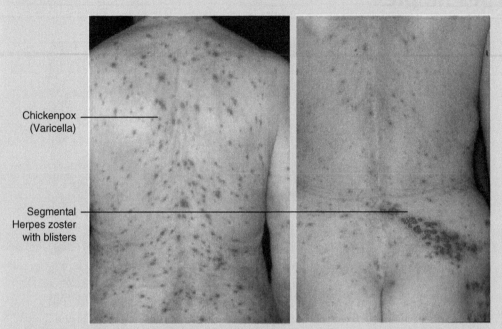

Chickenpox (Varicella)

Segmental Herpes zoster with blisters

Cl: Generalized papulovesicles and vesicles in different stages of development. Difference between varizella and herpes zoster is due to their clinical presentation.

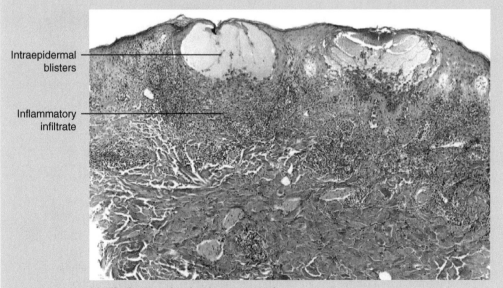

Intraepidermal blisters

Inflammatory infiltrate

Hi: Like herpes simplex (*see*, page 87).

DIFFERENTIAL DIAGNOSIS: **Poxvirus and other viral infections, ecthyma contagiosum (ORF)**

Tense blister

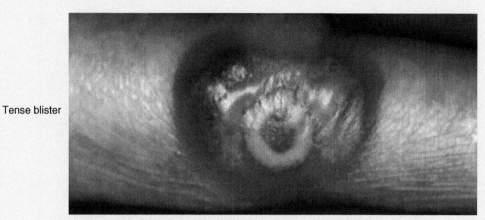

Cl: Solitary hemorrhagic blistering lesion usually on a finger.

Necrosis
and
hemorrhage

Ballooning of
epidermal cells

Blister with
eosinophils

Inflammatory
infiltrate with
eosinophils

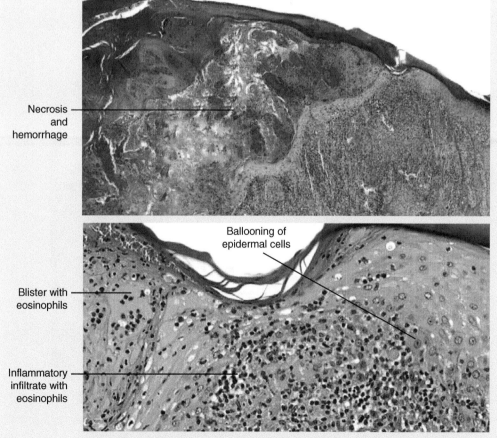

Hi: Epithelial hyperplasia, eosinophilic intracytoplasmic inclusions (Guarnieri bodies), mixed dermal infiltrate.

EPIDERMIS

DIFFERENTIAL DIAGNOSIS: Cytomegalovirus infection

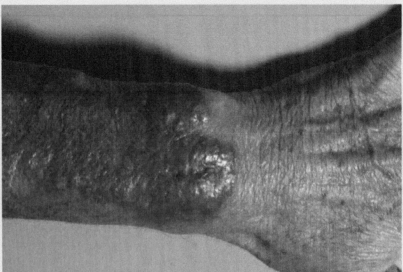

Erythema and blister formation

Cl: Variable depending on localization. Vesicular or superficial ulceration with crust.

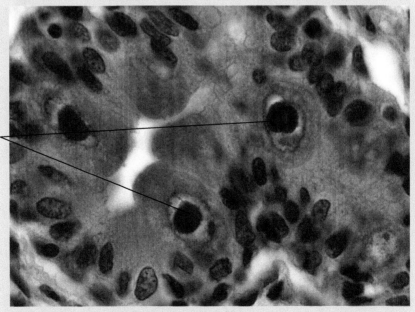

Owl eye cells (lung)

Hi: Endothelial cells with inclusions (owl eye cells) in the small dermal vessels (specimen from lung).

DIFFERENTIAL DIAGNOSIS: Hand, foot and mouth disease (Coxsackievirus)

Tiny erythematous blisters

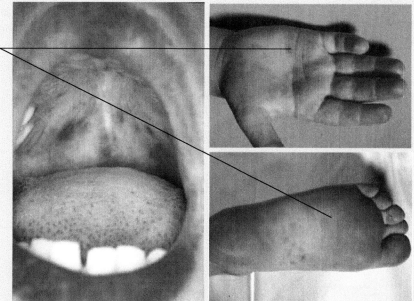

Cl: Tiny papulovesicles on palms and soles and on the palate.

Spongiotic vesicle

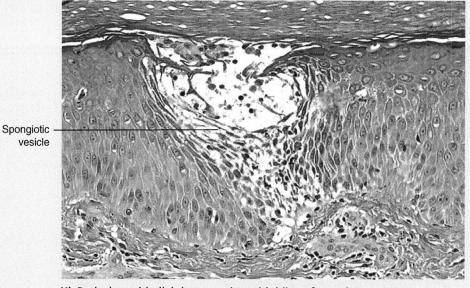

Hi: Reticular epithelial degeneration with blister formation.

Other Diagnosis

Pemphigus vulgaris (see Bullous, acantholytic, page 58*): Intraepidermal blister formation due to suprabasal acantholysis. No necrotic keratinocytes. No ballooning.*

Erythema multiforme: Interface changes, necrotic keratinocytes, edema in the upper dermis, no ballooning (see Necrotic, page 80*).*

Pityriasis lichenoides, acute: Interface changes, focal spongiosis, single necrotic keratinocytes and hyperparakeratosis with inclusions of neutrophils, no intraepidermal blister or vesicle formation (see page 84*).*

Comment

Differentiation between herpes simplex virus and varicella zoster virus is only possible by immunohisto-chemical, molecularbiologic or virological studies.

References

Boyd, A. S., J. P. Zwerner, and J. L. Miller (2012). "Herpes simplex virus-induced plasmacytic atypia." *J Cutan Pathol* **39**(2): 270–3.

Chisholm, C. and L. Lopez (2011). "Cutaneous infections caused by Herpesviridae: a review." *Arch Pathol Lab Med* **135**(10): 1357–62.

PROTOTYPE: **Verruca vulgaris**

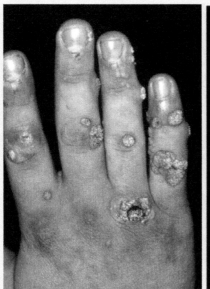 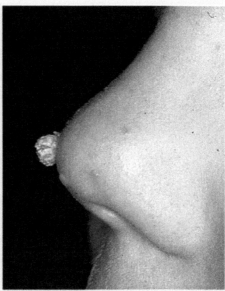

Cl: Solitary or grouped papules showing massive hyperkeratosis and sometimes significant inflammation.

Digitated epidermal hyperplasia

Papillomatosis

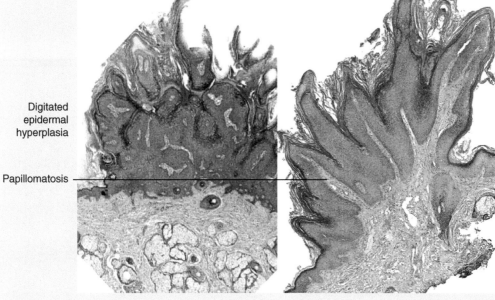

EPIDERMIS

EPIDERMIS

Verruca vulgaris

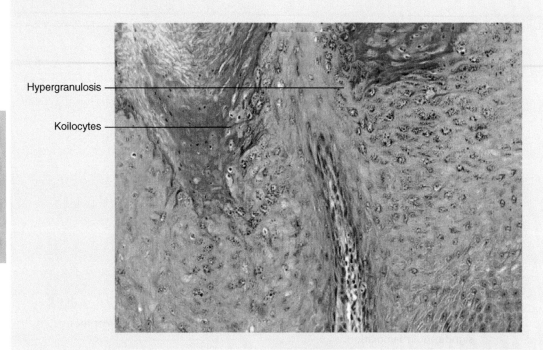

Hypergranulosis —

Koilocytes —

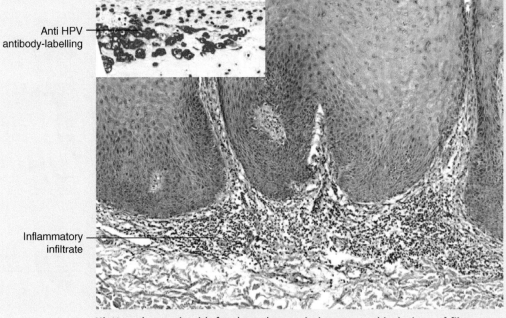

Anti HPV
antibody-labelling —

Inflammatory
infiltrate —

Hi: Hyperkeratosis with focal parakeratosis, intracorneal inclusions of fibrous hemorrhagic exsudate, digitated epidermal hyperplasia with koilocytes and confluent rete ridges, and papillomatosis, hypergranulosis with enlarged keratohyalin granules, dilated vessels in the papillary dermis.

VARIANT: **Verruca plana**

Flat brown
papules

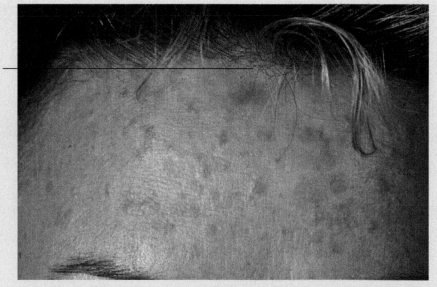

Cl: Hyperkeratotic (verruciform) papules.

Koilocytes

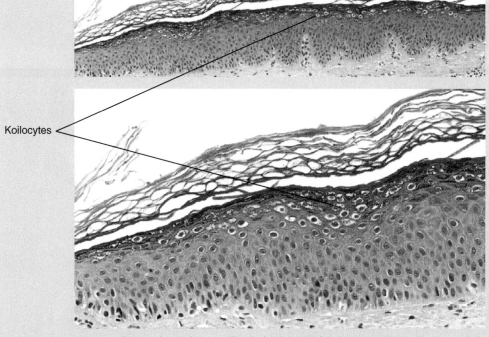

Hi: Hyperkeratosis, slight acanthosis, koilocytes (bird's eye cells) in the
granular layer.

EPIDERMIS

VARIANT: Condyloma acuminatum

Cauliflower-like proliferations

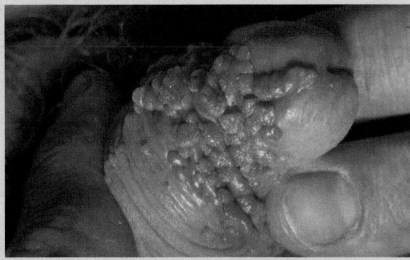

Cl: Papular and verruciforme lesions in anogenital localization.

Lack of hyperkeratosis

Acanthosis, papillomatosis,

Dilated vessels

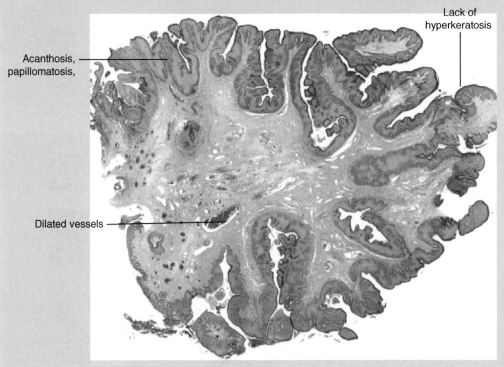

Hi: Acanthopapilloma with only a few koilocytes and focal hyperparakeratosis.

VARIANT: Bowenoid papulosis (Penile or vulvar intraepithelial neoplasia, grade 2 or 3)

Flat papules

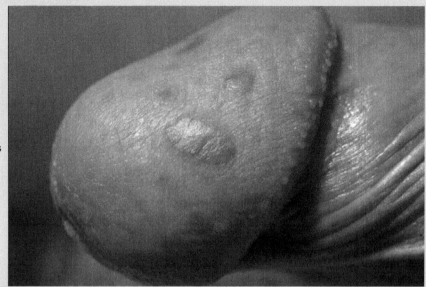

Cl: Solitary or confluent flat papular eruptions in anogenital localization.

Acanthosis, papillomatosis,

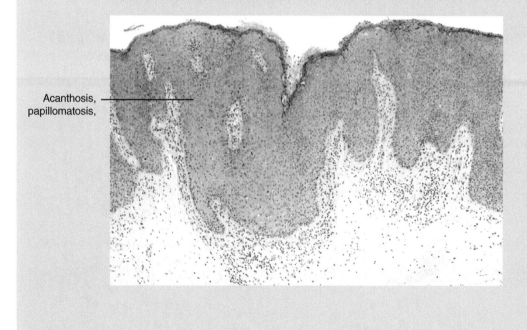

Bowenoid papulosis (Penile or vulvar intraepithelial neoplasia, grade 2 or 3)

EPIDERMIS

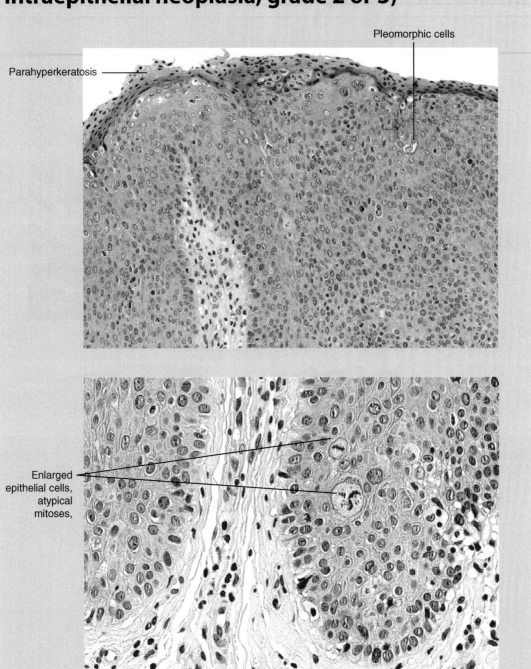

Hi: Atypical epithelial cells with nuclear pleomorphism and mitotic activity.

DIFFERENTIAL DIAGNOSIS: **Bowen's disease**

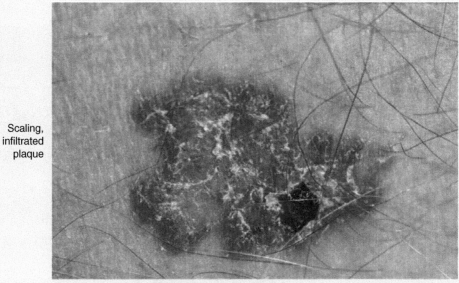

Scaling,
infiltrated
plaque

Cl: Circumscribed erythematous plaque with scaling or erosion and crust.

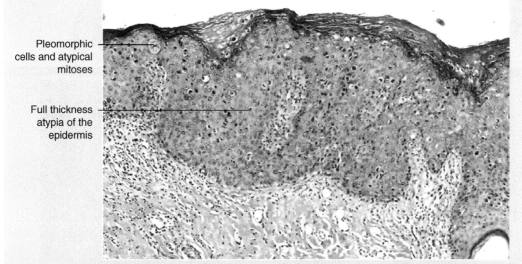

Pleomorphic
cells and atypical
mitoses

Full thickness
atypia of the
epidermis

Hi: Full thickness atypia of the epidermis, clumped and pleomorphic nuclei, mitoses.
Occasionally associated with HPV infection.

EPIDERMIS

DIFFERENTIAL DIAGNOSIS: Epidermodysplasia verruciformis (Lewandowsky-Lutz)

Brownish plaques on the dorsum of one hand

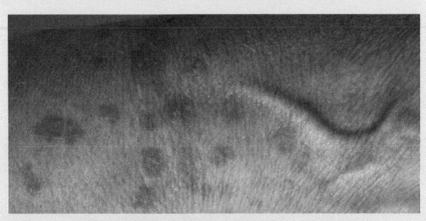

Cl: Genodermatosis, tiny circumscribed lesions, mostly on the extremities.

Verruciform acanthosis and papillomatosis

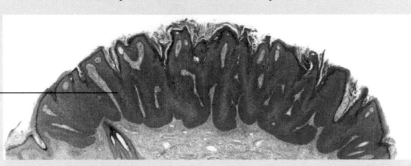

Typical «blue cells»

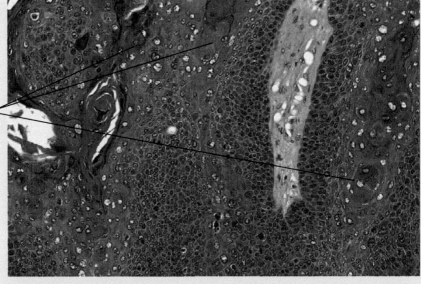

Hi: Intraepidermal enlarged keratinocytes with bluish cytoplasm ("blue cells"). Infection with beta/EV-HPV types.

DIFFERENTIAL DIAGNOSIS: **Seborrheic keratosis**

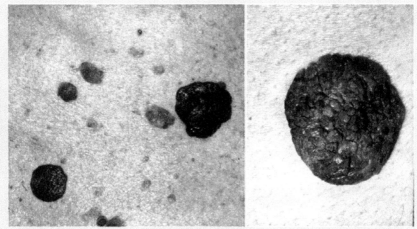

Keratotic papules and nodules of variable color

Cl: Various features. Usually brown to black irregularly hyperkeratotic papules or nodules.

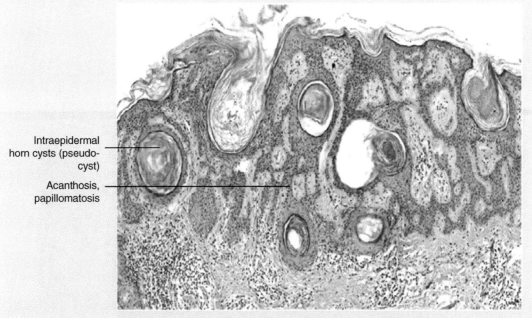

Intraepidermal horn cysts (pseudo-cyst)

Acanthosis, papillomatosis

Hi: Acanthoma with intraepidermal horn cysts, no koilocytes.

DIFFERENTIAL DIAGNOSIS: Verrucous epidermal nevus

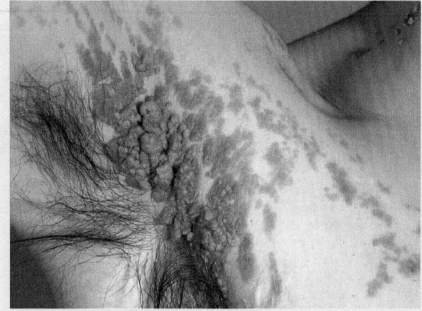

Lesions present since birth or early childhood

Cl: Present since early childhood.

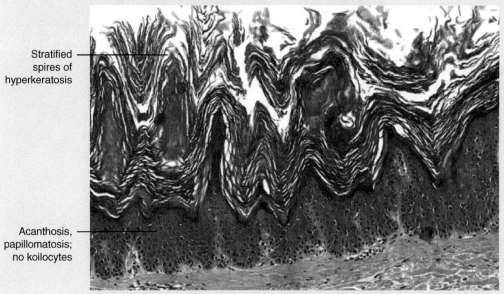

Stratified spires of hyperkeratosis

Acanthosis, papillomatosis; no koilocytes

Hi: Acanthosis, papillomatosis, hyperkeratosis, no koilocytes.

EPIDERMIS

Other Diagnosis

Focal oral hyperplasia (Heck's disease): large epithelial cells in the upper layers of the oral mucosa. Linked to HPV 13 and 32.

References

Requena, L. and C. Requena (2010). "[Histopathology of the more common viral skin infections]." *Actas Dermosifiliogr* **101**(3): 201–16.

Spielvogel, R. L., C. Austin, and A. B. Ackerman. (1983). "Inverted follicular keratosis is not a specific keratosis but a verruca vulgaris (or seborrheic keratosis) with squamous eddies." *Am J Dermatopathol* **5**(5): 427–42.

EPIDERMIS

PROTOTYPE: Chronic radiodermatitis

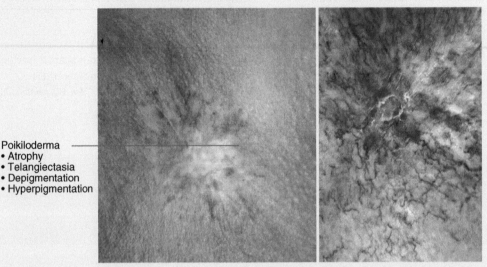

Poikiloderma
• Atrophy
• Telangiectasia
• Depigmentation
• Hyperpigmentation

Cl: Years after superficial (soft) or electron beam radiation. The skin shows atrophy with loss of rete ridges, hyper- and depigmentation and telangiectasias. This feature also is referred to as poikiloderma.

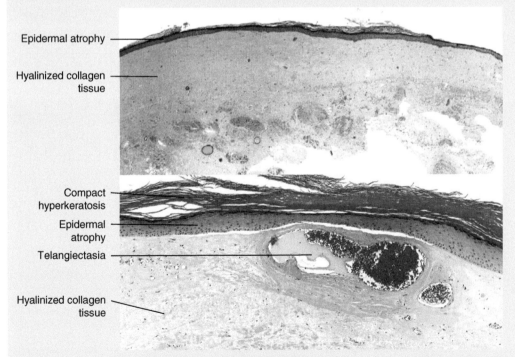

Epidermal atrophy

Hyalinized collagen tissue

Compact hyperkeratosis

Epidermal atrophy

Telangiectasia

Hyalinized collagen tissue

Hi: Atrophy of the epidermis, basal hyperpigmentation, hyalinized collagen tissue, telangiectatic vessels in the upper dermis, and melanophages.

DIFFERENTIAL DIAGNOSIS: Poikiloderma vasculare atrophicans Jacobi

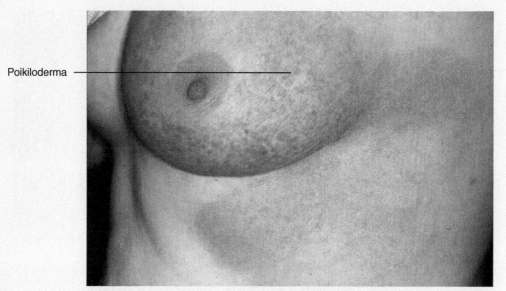

Poikiloderma

Cl: Mottled slightly scaling erythematous patches.

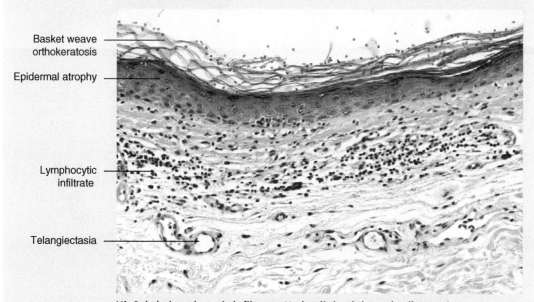

Basket weave orthokeratosis

Epidermal atrophy

Lymphocytic infiltrate

Telangiectasia

Hi: Subtle lymphocytic infiltrate. No hyalinized dermal collagen tissue.

EPIDERMIS

EPIDERMIS

DIFFERENTIAL DIAGNOSIS: Lichen sclerosus et atrophicus

Whitish atrophic plaque

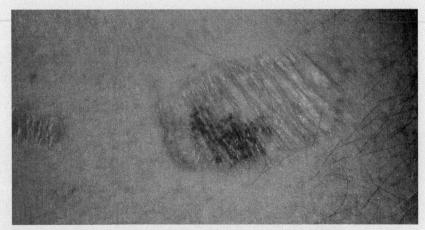

Cl: Whitish atrophic plaques; occasional intracutaneous bleeding, especially in the genital area.

Epidermal atrophy

Subepidermal hyalinized collagen tissue

Vertical streaks

Lymphocytic infiltrate

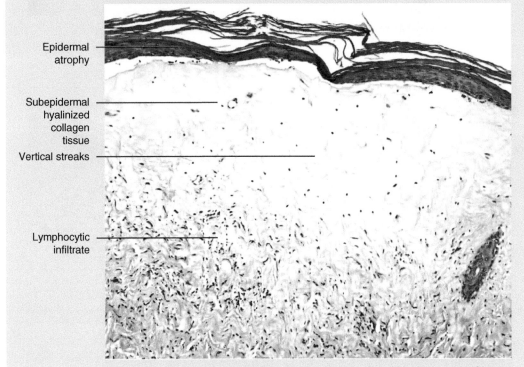

Hi: Initially and at the margins of the lesions there is a band-like lichenoid infiltrate, very similar to lichen planus (*see* page 110). Later there is a tricolor pattern in the center: atrophy of the (red) epidermis with hyperkeratosis, pale (white) hyalinized upper dermis with (blue) band-like infiltrate beneath the hyaline zone.

DIFFERENTIAL DIAGNOSIS: **Acrodermatitis chronica atrophicans**

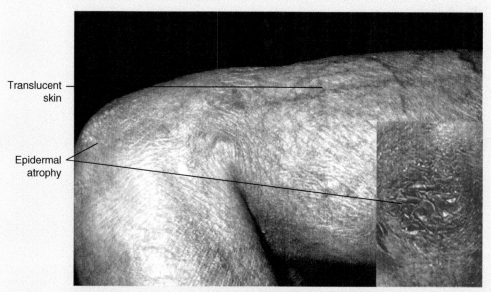

Translucent skin

Epidermal atrophy

Cl: Atrophy of the skin with translucent superficial vessels.

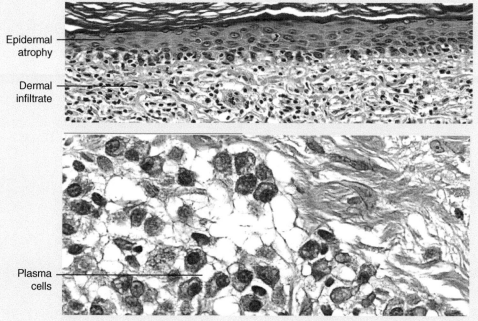

Epidermal atrophy

Dermal infiltrate

Plasma cells

Hi: Perivascular infiltrates with numerous plasma cells. Atrophy of the epidermis and dermis in fully developed stage.

Other Diagnosis

Morphea: Thickened collagen bundles, broadened dermis and subcutaneous septa. Sweat glands engulfed by compact collagen bundles (see Chapter 4, Sclerosis, page 205*).*

Scar: Fibrotic collagen tissue with loss of elastic fibers.

CHAPTER 3

Dermal–epidermal Junction (Interface)

<table>
<tr><td>CHAPTER MENU</td></tr>
<tr><td>Lichenoid
Subepidermal blistering</td></tr>
</table>

Atlas of Dermatopathology: Practical Differential Diagnosis by Clinicopathologic Pattern, First Edition.
Edited by Günter Burg MD, Werner Kempf MD, and Heinz Kutzner MD. Co-Editors: Josef Feit MD, and Laszlo Karai MD.
© 2015 John Wiley & Sons, Ltd. Published 2015 by John Wiley & Sons, Ltd.

PROTOTYPE: Lichen (ruber) planus

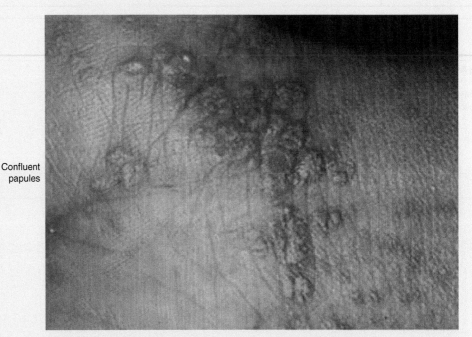

Confluent papules

Cl: Pruritic polygonal violet papules, mucosa with Wickham striae.

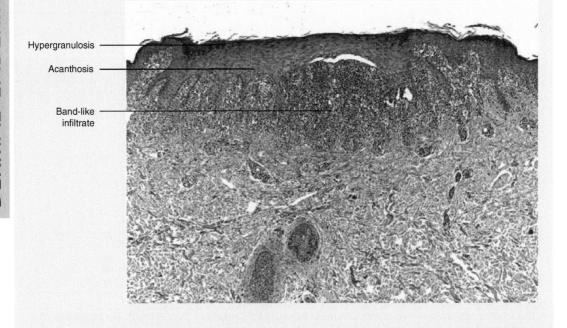

Hypergranulosis

Acanthosis

Band-like infiltrate

Lichen planus

Hypergranulosis

Saw tooth-
like elongation
of rete ridges

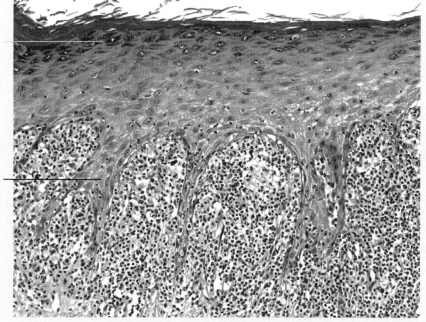

Vacuolization, obscuring of the interface and focal cleft formation

Hypergranulosis

Civatte body

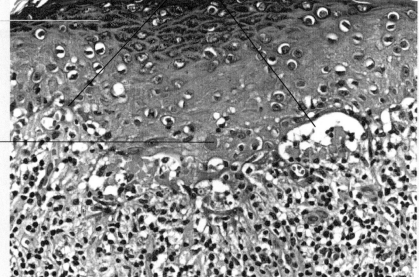

Hi: Interface dermatitis, acanthosis, V-shaped hypergranulosis, hyperkeratosis, subepidermal band-like lymphocytic infiltrate.

DERMAL–EPIDERMAL JUNCTION (INTERFACE)

DERMAL–EPIDERMAL JUNCTION (INTERFACE)

VARIANT: Hypertrophic (syn: verrucous) lichen planus

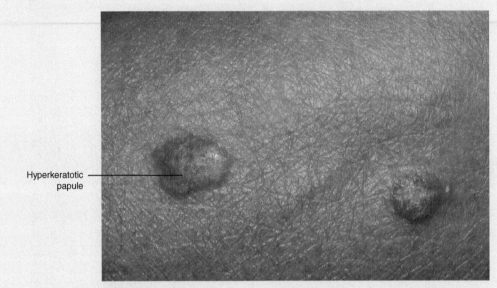

Hyperkeratotic papule

Cl: Verrucous papules.

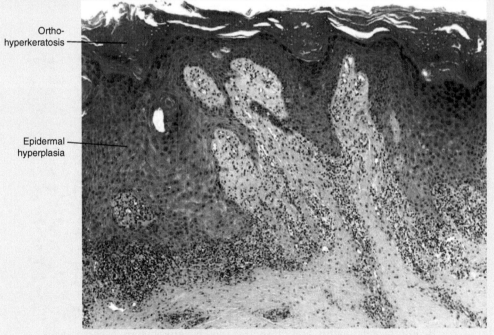

Ortho-hyperkeratosis

Epidermal hyperplasia

Hi: Orthohyperkeratosis, pseudocarcinomatous hyperplasia, interface lymphocytic infiltrate.

DIFFERENTIAL DIAGNOSIS: Lichenoid drug reaction

Maculo-papular lesions

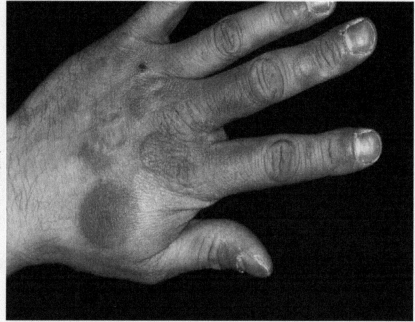

Cl: Disseminated maculo-papular lesions.

Apoptotic keratinocytes

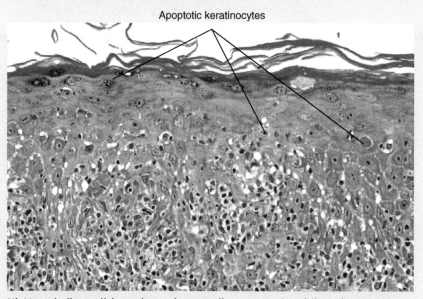

Hi: Very similar to lichen planus, but usually many eosinophils and apoptotic keratinocytes, occasionally parakeratosis.

DERMAL–EPIDERMAL JUNCTION (INTERFACE)

DERMAL–EPIDERMAL JUNCTION (INTERFACE)

DIFFERENTIAL DIAGNOSIS: Lichen nitidus

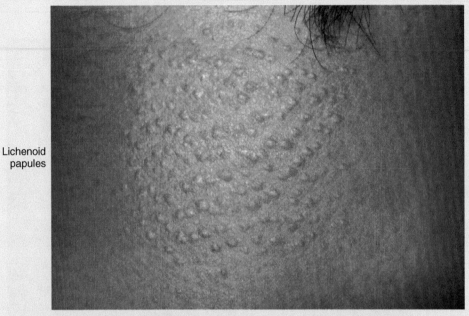

Lichenoid
papules

Cl: Group of tiny papules.

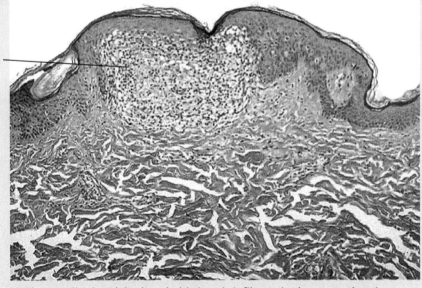

Lymphohistiocytic
infiltrate in the
papillary dermis

Hi: Circumscribed nodular lymphohistiocytic infiltrate in the upper dermis.

DIFFERENTIAL DIAGNOSIS: Lichen aureus

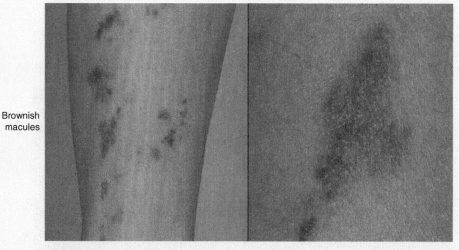

Brownish macules

CI: *Red-brown* circumscribed lesion.

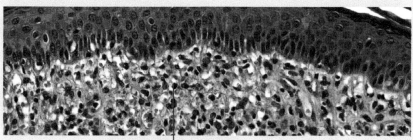

Erythrocyte extravasation   Hemosiderin (Prussian blue)

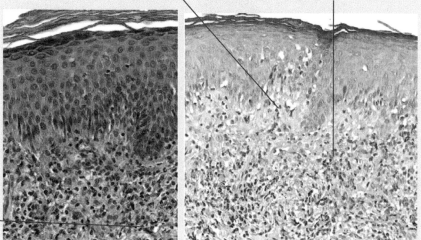

Hemosiderin

Hi: Band-like infiltrate, less pronounced vacuolization, extravasated erythrocytes, hemosiderin deposits.

DERMAL–EPIDERMAL JUNCTION (INTERFACE)

DIFFERENTIAL DIAGNOSIS: Acute graft-versus-host reaction

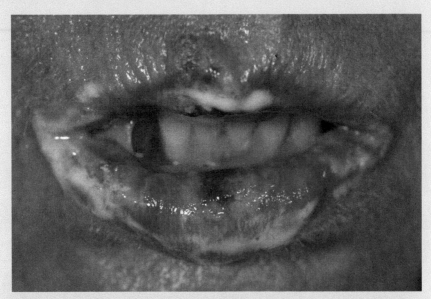

Cl: Massive necrolytic changes of the oral mucosa, similar to drug induced toxic epidermal necrolysis (TEN, *see* page 78) in a patient with prior bone marrow transplantation.

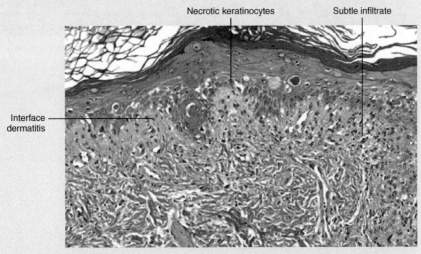

Hi: Thinned epidermis, numerous apoptotic keratinocytes, satellite cell necrosis, vacuolar change at the dermal–epidermal junction, less intense lymphocytic infiltrate.

DERMAL–EPIDERMAL JUNCTION (INTERFACE)

DIFFERENTIAL DIAGNOSIS: Lupus erythematosus, acute systemic

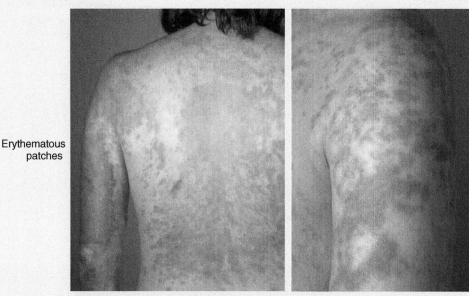

Erythematous patches

Cl: Patchy bizarre and confluent erythemas.

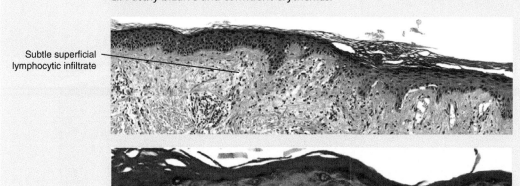

Subtle superficial lymphocytic infiltrate

Interface dermatitis

DERMAL–EPIDERMAL JUNCTION (INTERFACE)

Lupus erythematosus

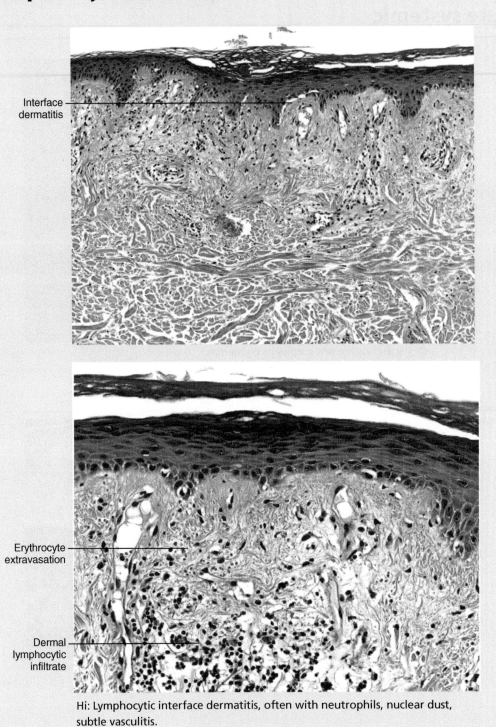

Interface dermatitis

Erythrocyte extravasation

Dermal lymphocytic infiltrate

Hi: Lymphocytic interface dermatitis, often with neutrophils, nuclear dust, subtle vasculitis.

DIFFERENTIAL DIAGNOSIS: Dermatomyositis

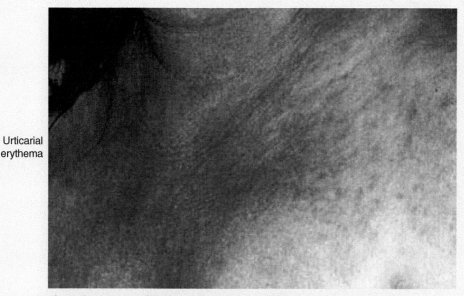

Urticarial erythema

Cl: Erythema or poikilodermatic lesions or Gottron papules on fingers.

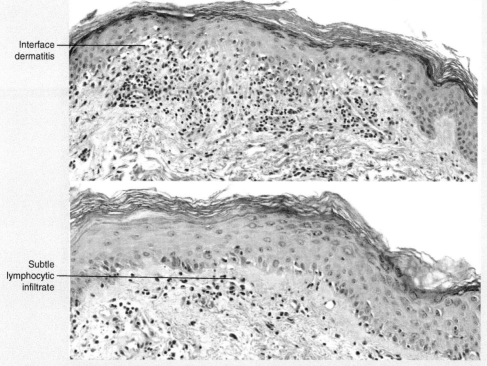

Interface dermatitis

Subtle lymphocytic infiltrate

Hi: Interface dermatitis, deposits of mucin in the upper dermis, sparse perivascular infiltrate.

DERMAL–EPIDERMAL JUNCTION (INTERFACE)

DIFFERENTIAL DIAGNOSIS: Mycosis fungoides (early stage)

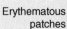

Erythematous patches

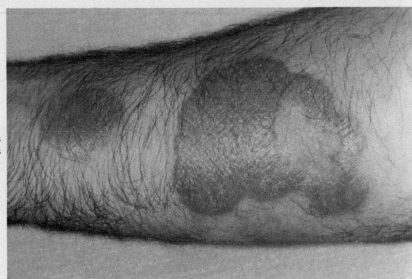

Cl: Longstanding patches.

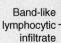

Band-like lymphocytic infiltrate

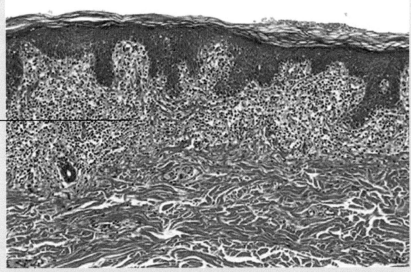

Hi: Lining-up of atypical lymphocytes along the dermal–epidermal junction, rather subtle epidermotropism without spongiosis. Infiltrate may be band-like, but rarely with associated necrotic keratinocytes.

Other Diagnosis

Lichen planus-like keratosis: Solitary lesion. Predilection site: chest. Histology is identical to lichen planus, in the margins often hyperpigmented elongated rete ridges.

Keratosis lichenoides chronica: Hyperkeratotic flat papules, preferentially on the extremities, often in linear arrangement. Histology shows acanthosis, orthohyperkeratosis, interface dermatitis, lichenoid infiltrate in the upper dermis.

Pityriasis lichenoides et varioliformis acuta (PLEVA): (see Chapter 2, Necrotic, page 84): Disseminated red scaly maculo-papular lesions. Focal vacuolization, spongiosis and hyperparakeratosis with inclusions of neutrophils, wedge-shaped superficial and deep lymphocytic infiltrate.

Fixed drug eruption (see Chapter 2, Edema, page 81): Usually solitary circumscribed brownish patch, recurrence after intake of the drug. Histologically there is incontinence of pigment. Apoptotic keratinocytes in all epidermal layers, eosinophils and occasionally neutrophils.

References

Akasu, R., L. From, and H. J. Kahn (1993). "Lymphocyte and macrophage subsets in active and inactive lesions of lichen planus." *Am J Dermatopathol* **15**(3): 217–23.

Aung, P. P., J. Burns S, and J. Bhawan. (2014). "Lichen aureus: An unusual histopathological presentation: A case report and a review of literature." *Am J Dermatopathol* **36**(1): e1–4.

Camacho, D., U. Pielasinski, J. M. Revelles, *et al.* (2011). "Lichen scrofulosorum mimicking lichen planus." *Am J Dermatopathol* **33**(2): 186–91.

Citarella, L., C. Massone, H. Kerl, and L. Cerroni (2003). "Lichen sclerosus with histopathologic features simulating early mycosis fungoides." *Am J Dermatopathol* **25**(6): 463–5.

De Eusebio Murillo, E., E. Sanchez Yus, *et al.* (1999). "Lichen nitidus of the palms: a case with peculiar histopathologic features." *Am J Dermatopathol* **21**(2): 161–4.

Gomes, M. A., M. J. Staquet, and J. Thivolet (1981). "Staining of colloid bodies by keratin antisera in lichen planus." *Am J Dermatopathol* **3**(4): 341–7.

LeBoit, P. E. (2000). "A thickened basement membrane is a clue to...lichen sclerosus!" *Am J Dermatopathol* **22**(5): 457–8.

Ragaz, A. and A. B. Ackerman (1981). "Evolution, maturation, and regression of lesions of lichen planus. New observations and correlations of clinical and histologic findings." *Am J Dermatopathol* **3**(1): 5–25.

Roustan, G., M. Hospital, C. Villegas, *et al.* (1994). "Lichen planus with predominant plasma cell infiltrate." *Am J Dermatopathol* **16**(3): 311–14.

PROTOTYPE: **Bullous pemphigoid**

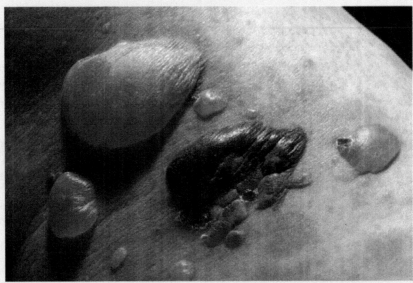

Tense bullae, some hemorrhage

Cl: Initially erythematous and urticarial patches and plaques (prebullous stage), marked pruritus; later tense, sometimes hemorrhagic blisters; mucosal involvement possible.

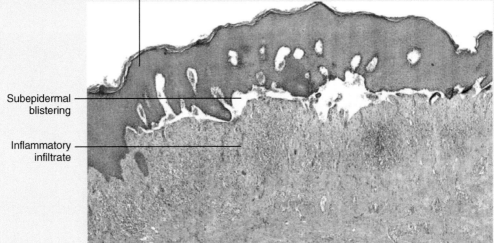

Thick roof of the bulla

Subepidermal blistering

Inflammatory infiltrate

Hi: Clear-cut cleft or bulla at the dermal-epidermal junction. Associated eosinophilic infiltrate.

Bullous pemphigoid

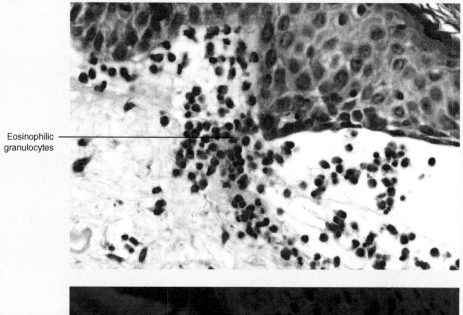

Eosinophilic granulocytes

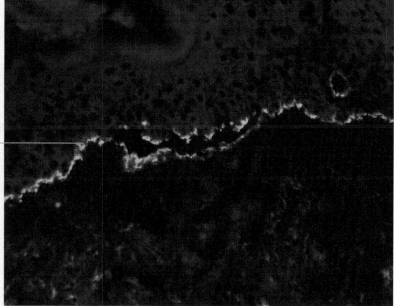

DIF: linear deposition of antibodies (IgG, C3)

Hi: Subepidermal blister, eosinophils and neutrophils in the blister cavity and in the dermal infiltrate, no necrotic keratinocytes, no significant edema in the dermis, admixture of plasma cells. Subepidermal blistering is lacking in the prebullous state. Immunohistochemistry: Linear deposits of C3d at the junctional zone. Direct immunofluorescence: Linear IgG and C3 deposits at the junctional zone of adjacent non-lesional skin or mucosa.

DERMAL–EPIDERMAL JUNCTION (INTERFACE)

Bullous pemphigoid, early urticarial stage

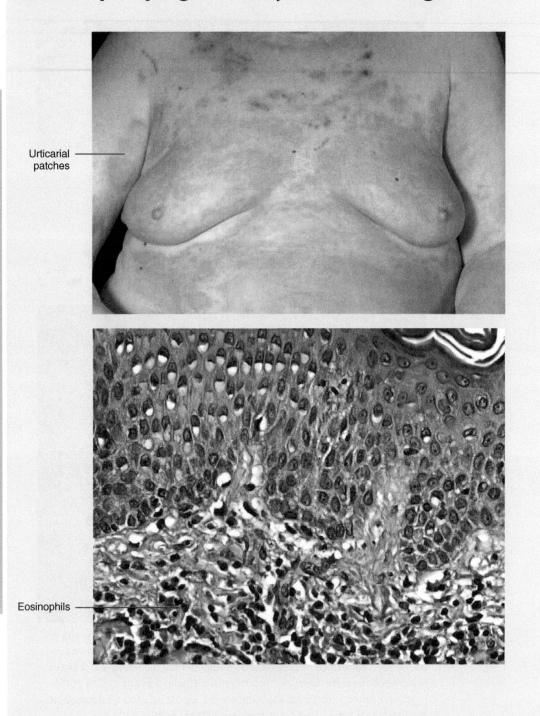

Urticarial patches

Eosinophils

DIFFERENTIAL DIAGNOSIS: Autoimmune bullous disorders: Epidermolysis bullosa

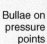

Bullae on pressure points

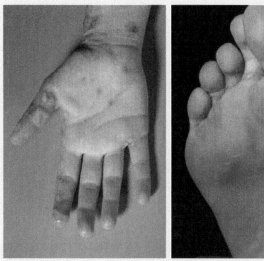

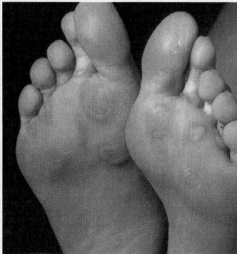

Cl: Epidermolysis bullosa simplex (Weber-Cockayne). Variable clinical features with mechanobullous blister formation.

Antibodies against collagen IV on the roof of the blister

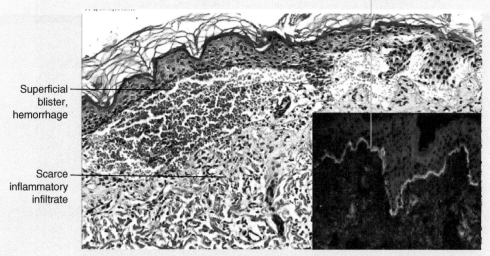

Superficial blister, hemorrhage

Scarce inflammatory infiltrate

Hi: Epidermolysis bullosa acquisita. Few inflammatory cells, split skin test and collagen IV staining (inset): antibodies on the roof of the blister.

DERMAL–EPIDERMAL JUNCTION (INTERFACE)

DIFFERENTIAL DIAGNOSIS: Pemphigoid gestationis

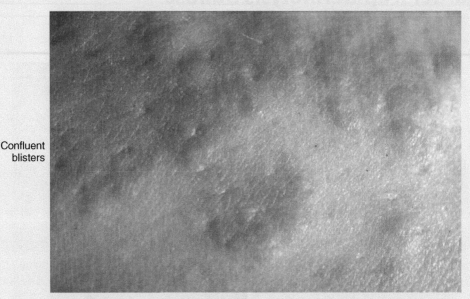

Confluent blisters

Cl: Pruritic papules and plaques, usually starting in the 3rd trimester of gestation in the abdominal region at any time during pregnancy or thereafter.

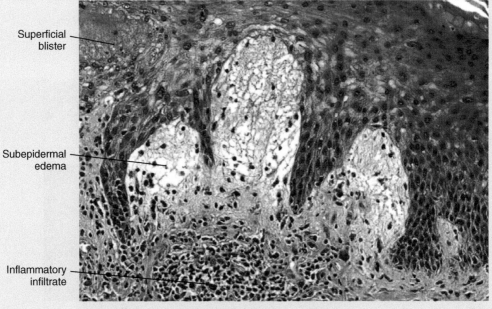

Superficial blister

Subepidermal edema

Inflammatory infiltrate

Hi: Histology and DIF identical to bullous pemphigoid.

DIFFERENTIAL DIAGNOSIS: Dermatitis herpetiformis (Duhring's disease)

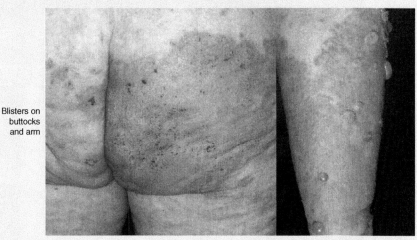

Blisters on buttocks and arm

Cl: Polymorphous (eczematous papules, plaques and vesicles) itching lesions, preferentially on elbows, knees and buttocks.

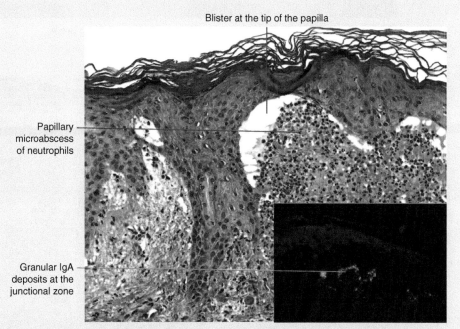

Blister at the tip of the papilla

Papillary microabscess of neutrophils

Granular IgA deposits at the junctional zone

Hi: Papillary microabscesses of neutrophils (and eosinophils). DIF (inset): Granular IgA deposits at the junctional zone.

IgA linear bullous dermatosis (see Chapter 2, Bullous, acantholytic, page 63): Pruritic erythematous papules and plaques, transforming into tense blisters in an annular or herpetiform arrangement. Histology shows infiltrates of neutrophils and eosinophils. DIF: linear IgA deposits along the junctional zone.

Systemic lupus erythematosus: urticarial lesions with band-like subepidermal neutrophilic infiltrate (see page 117).

Epidermolysis bullosa acquisita: bullous lesions with band-like subepidermal neutrophilic infiltrate.

Vancomycin-induced bullous dermatitis with band-like subepidermal neutrophilic infiltrate.

DERMAL–EPIDERMAL JUNCTION (INTERFACE)

DERMAL–EPIDERMAL JUNCTION (INTERFACE)

OTHER SKIN DISEASES: Porphyria cutanea tarda

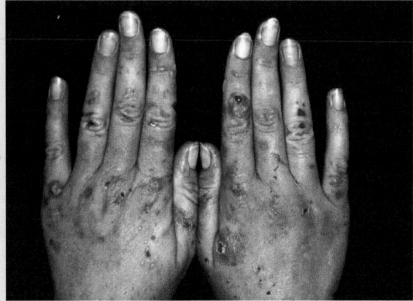

Small blisters, erosions, crusts

Cl: tense blisters, erosions with crust formation in sun exposed areas, preferentially back of the hands.

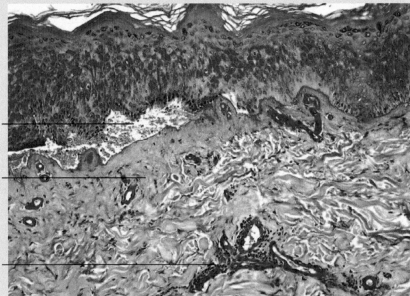

PAS stain:

Subepidermal blister

Fibrosis, lack of inflammation

Thickened vessel walls

Hi: Subepidermal blister, preserved papillae (festooning), almost no inflammatory infiltrate, thickening of vessel walls (PAS). Fibrosis.

OTHER SKIN DISEASES: Arthropod bite reaction

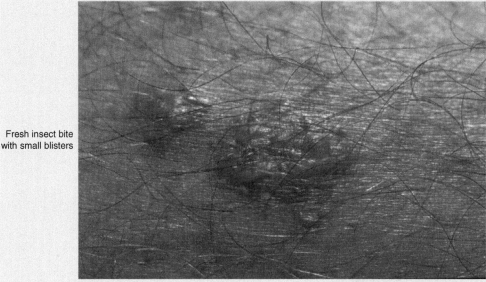

Fresh insect bite with small blisters

Cl: circumscribed urticarial wheal.

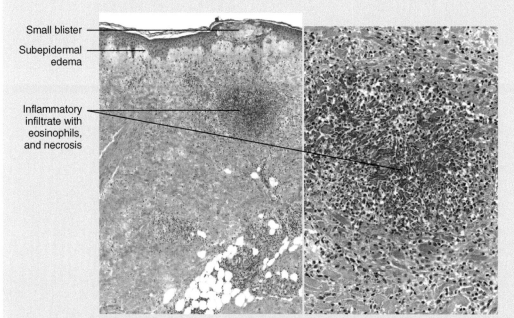

Small blister
Subepidermal edema

Inflammatory infiltrate with eosinophils, and necrosis

Hi: focal spongiosis, subepidermal edema, wedge-shaped infiltrate with eosinophils and neutrophils.

DERMAL–EPIDERMAL JUNCTION (INTERFACE)

OTHER SKIN DISEASES: Thermic or mechanical blistering

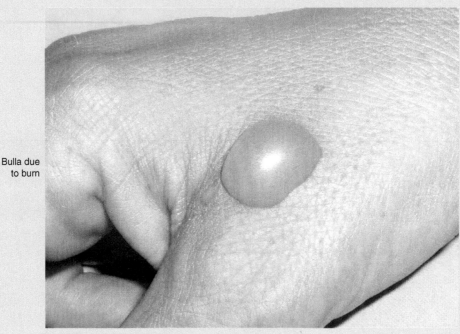

Bulla due to burn

Cl: Tense blister.

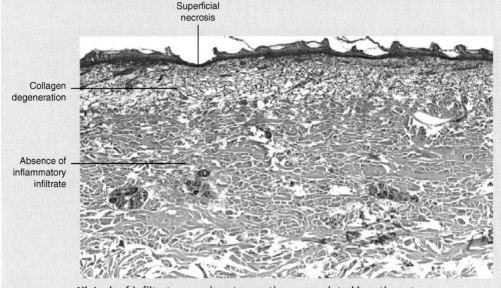

Superficial necrosis

Collagen degeneration

Absence of inflammatory infiltrate

Hi: Lack of infiltrate, prominent necrotic or vacuolated keratinocytes.

OTHER SKIN DISEASES: **Bullous drug eruption**

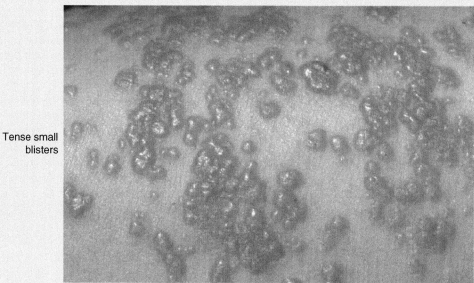

Tense small
blisters

Cl: Tense blisters on erythema.

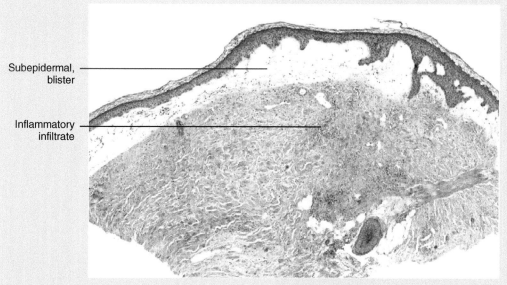

Subepidermal,
blister

Inflammatory
infiltrate

Hi: Subepidermal blister formation, necrotic keratinocytes, lymphocytic infiltrate
with eosinophils.

DERMAL–EPIDERMAL JUNCTION (INTERFACE)

Erythema (exsudativum) multiforme (see Chapter 2, Necrobiotic, page 80): *interface dermatitis, necrotic keratinocytes in all epidermal layers. Edema in upper dermis, lymphocytic infiltrate.*

References

Andrachuk, L., D. Ghazarian, S. Siddha, AND a. Al Habeeb. (2012). "Linear arrangement of neutrophils along the Basal layer in bullous pemphigoid: a unique histological finding." *Am J Dermatopathol* **34**(2): 192–3.

Barnadas, M. A., R. M. Pujol, R. Curell, *et al.* (2000). "Generalized pruritic eruption with suprabasal acantholysis preceeding the development of bullous pemphigoid." *J Cutan Pathol* **27**(2): 96–8.

Blenkinsopp, W. K., G. P. Haffenden, L. Fry, *et al.* (1983). "Histology of linear IgA disease, dermatitis herpetiformis, and bullous pemphigoid." *Am J Dermatopathol* **5**(6): 547–54.

Fisler, R. E., M. Saeb, M. G. Liang, *et al.* (2003). "Childhood bullous pemphigoid: A clinicopathologic study and review of the literature." *Am J Dermatopathol* **25**(3): 183–9.

Kneisel, A. and M. Hertl (2011). "Autoimmune bullous skin diseases. Part 2: diagnosis and therapy." *J Dtsch Dermatol Ges* **9**(11): 927–47.

Smolle, J. and H. Kerl (1984). "Pitfalls in the diagnosis of pemphigus vulgaris (early pemphigus vulgaris with features of bullous pemphigoid)." *Am J Dermatopathol* **6**(5): 429–35.

CHAPTER 4

Dermis

Atlas of Dermatopathology: Practical Differential Diagnosis by Clinicopathologic Pattern, First Edition.
Edited by Günter Burg MD, Werner Kempf MD, and Heinz Kutzner MD. Co-Editors: Josef Feit MD, and Laszlo Karai MD.
© 2015 John Wiley & Sons, Ltd. Published 2015 by John Wiley & Sons, Ltd.

PROTOTYPE: **Urticaria**

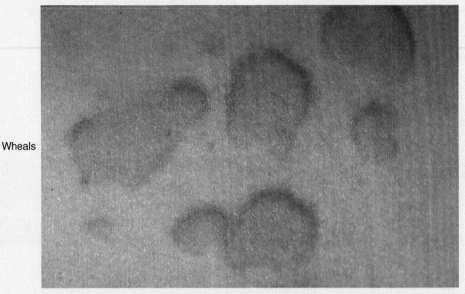

Wheals

Cl: Pruritic, transitory (usually a few hours), erythematous, slightly elevated plaques and patches with various pathogenetic background.

Sparse lymphocytic infiltrate with eosinophils

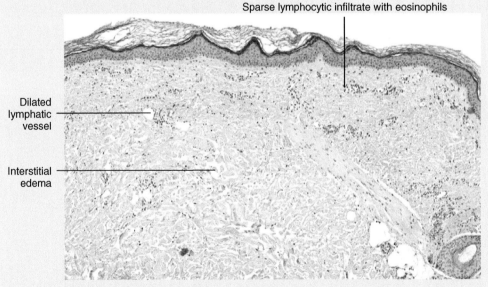

Dilated lymphatic vessel

Interstitial edema

Hi: Sparse inflammatory infiltrate. Histological clue: few granulocytes within vessel lumina and with interstitial splaying throughout the dermis.

Urticaria

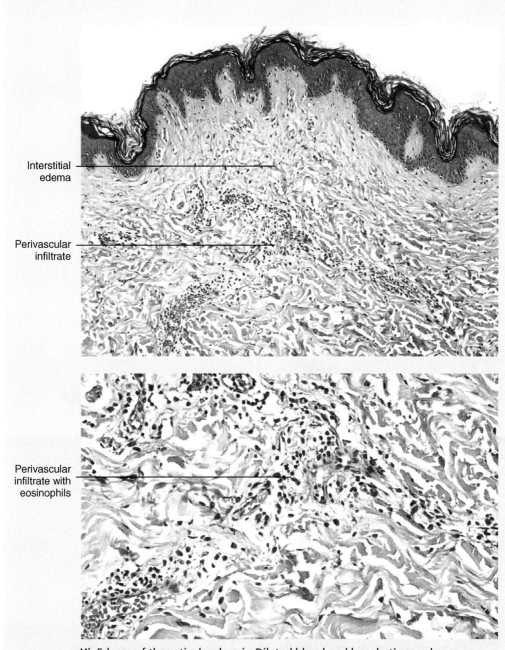

Interstitial edema

Perivascular infiltrate

Perivascular infiltrate with eosinophils

Hi: Edema of the reticular dermis. Dilated blood and lymphatic vessels, sparse perivascular and interstitial inflammatory infiltrate composed of eosinophils, neutrophils and lymphocytes. No epidermal changes.

DERMIS

DIFFERENTIAL DIAGNOSIS: Urticarial vasculitis

Urticaria

Cl: Urticarial lesions with purpura, which persists longer than 24 hours.

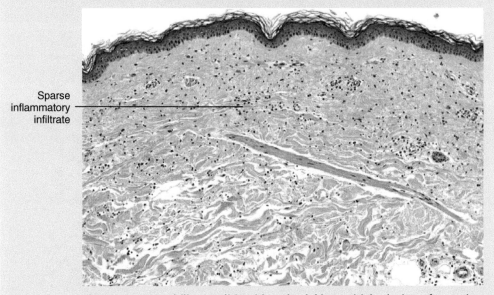

Sparse
inflammatory
infiltrate

Hi: Sparse neutrophilic vasculitis with urticarial interstitial splaying of granulocytes.

Urticarial vasculitis

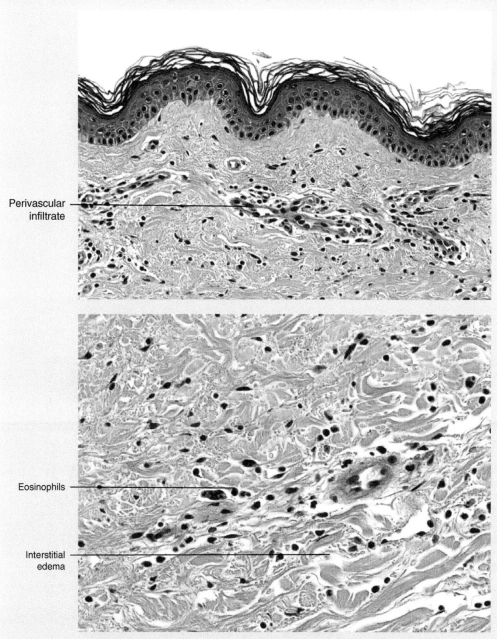

Perivascular
infiltrate

Eosinophils

Interstitial
edema

Hi: Infiltration of vessel walls of small dermal vessels by eosinophils and
neutrophils, nuclear dust.

DERMIS

DIFFERENTIAL DIAGNOSIS: Drug eruption (*see also* Chapter 2, Necrotic and Chapter 3, Lichenoid)

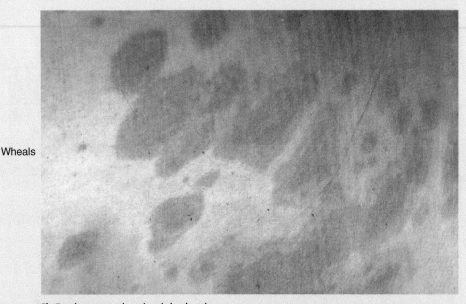

Wheals

Cl: Erythema and urticarial wheals.

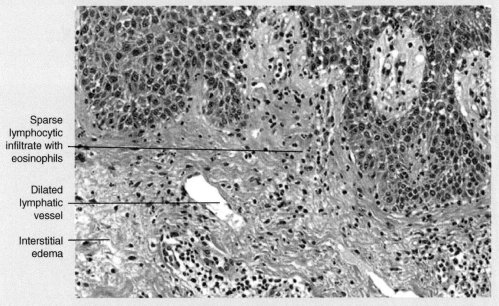

Sparse lymphocytic infiltrate with eosinophils

Dilated lymphatic vessel

Interstitial edema

Hi: Histology may be identical to urticaria. Occasionally interface changes. Clinically, mostly exanthema with maculo-papular lesions.

DIFFERENTIAL DIAGNOSIS: Pruritic urticarial papules and plaques of pregnancy

Confluent
urticarial
papules

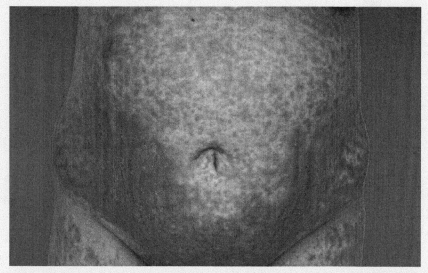

Cl: Pruritic urticarial papules and plaques usually occurring on the abdomen in the last trimester of pregnancy.

Perivascular
lymphocytic
infiltrate

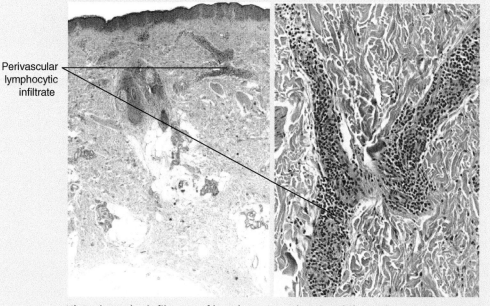

Hi: Perivascular infiltrates of lymphocytes and eosinophils. Epidermal changes with spongiosis may be present.

DERMIS

DIFFERENTIAL DIAGNOSIS: Lymphedema

Massive lymphedema congenital (left) and acquired (right)

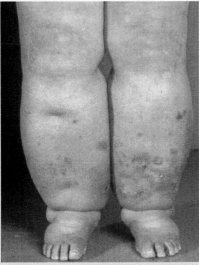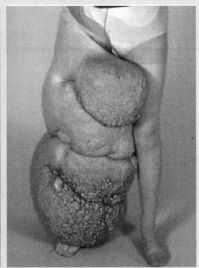

Cl: Swelling usually on the lower legs or in areas of blocked lymph drainage.

Edema and fibrosis

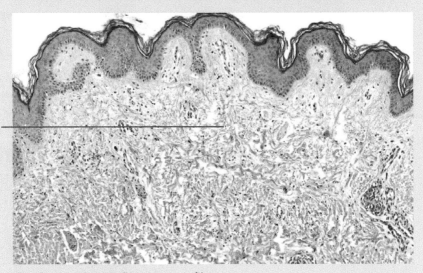

Hi: Edema without inflammatory infiltrate.

Other Diagnosis

Neutrophilic urticaria: Perivascular infiltrate in the upper and mid dermis with predominance of neutrophils. May be associated with Schnitzler syndrome (rare multisystem disorder with urticaria and monoclonal gammopathy).

Mastocytosis (Urticaria pigmentosa): Subtle perivascular infiltrate with admixture of eosinophils and numerous mast cells (>20 mast cells per HPF).

Erysipelas (*see* Non-granulomatous, neutrophil- or eosinophil-rich, page 162): *Perivascular and interstitial infiltrate with predominance of neutrophils. Edema. Clinically circumscribed erythema and fever.*

Bullous pemphigoid, prebullous phase (*see* Non-granulomatous, neutrophil- or eosinophil-rich, page 166): *Clinically and histologically simulating urticaria with dermal infiltrates of eosinophils.*

Dermatitis herpetiformis (Duhring) (*see* Chapter 3, Subepidermal blistering, page 127): *Accumulations of neutrophils and vacuolization in the papillae.*

Arthropod bite reaction (*see also* Chapter 3, Subepidermal blistering, page 129): *Wedge-shaped infiltrate with lymphocytes and eosinophils. Epidermis with focal spongiosis.*

References

Jordaan, H. F. and J. W. Schneider (1997). "Papular urticaria: a histopathologic study of 30 patients." Am J Dermatopathol **19**(2): 119–26.

Kossard, S., I. Hamann, and B. Wilkinson (2006). "Defining urticarial dermatitis: a subset of dermal hypersensitivity reaction pattern." *Arch Dermatol* **142**(1): 29–34.

Sanchez, J. L. and O. Benmaman (1992). "Clinicopathological correlation in chronic urticaria." *Am J Dermatopathol* **14**(3): 220–3.

Stewart, G. E., 2nd (2002). "Histopathology of chronic urticaria." *Clin Rev Allergy Immunol* **23**(2): 195–200.

Toyoda, M., T. Maruyama, and J. Bhawan (1996). "Free eosinophil granules in urticaria: a correlation with the duration of wheals." *Am J Dermatopathol* **18**(1): 49–57.

PROTOTYPE: Lupus erythematosus (LE), chronic discoid

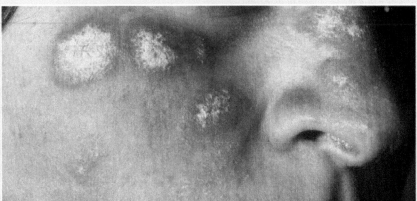

Disk shaped erythematous hyperkeratotic plaques

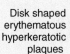

Cl: Coin or disk-shaped erythematous plaques with follicular hyperkeratoses and a tendency to heal with scarring, usually on light-exposed areas.

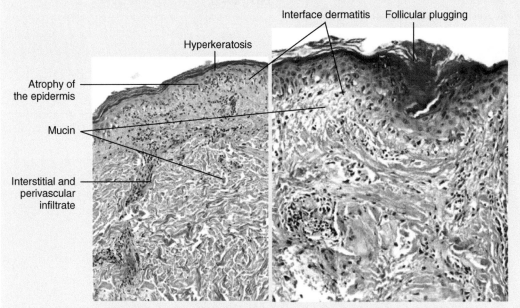

Interface dermatitis   Follicular plugging

Hyperkeratosis

Atrophy of the epidermis

Mucin

Interstitial and perivascular infiltrate

Hi: Hyperkeratosis, follicular plugs. Atrophy of the epidermis, apoptotic keratinocytes. Vacuolization of the junctional zone (interface dermatitis). Patchy or cuff-like perivascular and periadnexal dense lymphocytic infiltrates. No eosinophils. Interstitial mucin in all levels of the dermis.

VARIANT: Systemic LE (SLE)

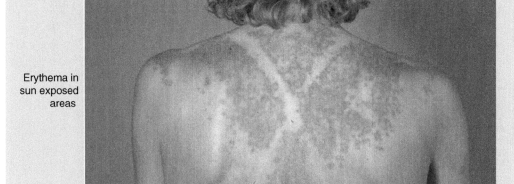

Erythema in sun exposed areas

Cl: The diagnosis is based on 4 or more ACR (American College of Rheumatology) criteria being fulfilled. These include: "butterfly" erythema of the face, photosensitive erythematous diffuse macules, oral ulcerations.

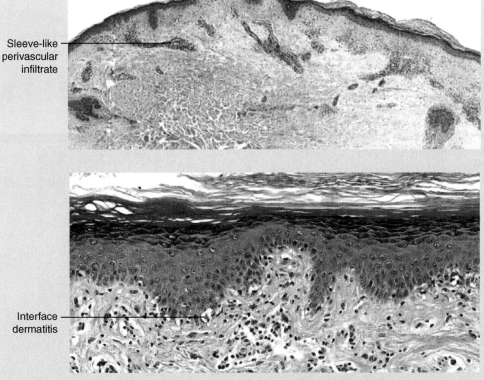

Sleeve-like perivascular infiltrate

Interface dermatitis

Hi: Interface dermatitis, necrotic keratinocytes, sparse inflammatory infiltrate. Edema and mucin in the upper dermis.

DERMIS

VARIANT: Subacute cutaneous LE (SCLE)

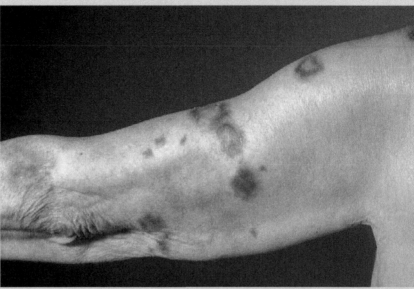

Annular erythematous lesions

Cl: Non-scarring, polycyclic-annular or papulosquamous (psoriasiform) plaques which usually involve the upper half of the body and are clearly UV light-provoked. If present, systemic symptoms (arthritis, fever, malaise) are milder than in SLE (severe CNS or renal disease rare).

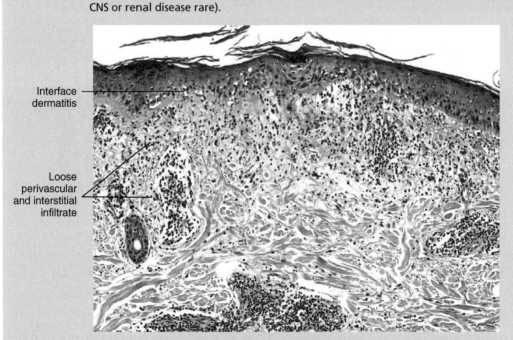

Interface dermatitis

Loose perivascular and interstitial infiltrate

Hi: Interface dermatitis. Necrotic keratinocytes may be present. Perivascular lymphocytic infiltrate in the upper dermis, more prominent than in systemic LE. Dermal mucin.

VARIANT: LE tumidus

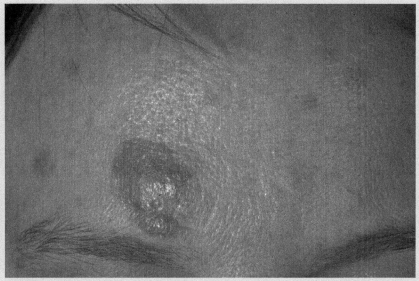

Nodular lesions on the forehead

Cl: Papulo-nodular lesions or plaques without scaling. Face and trunk are preferential localizations.

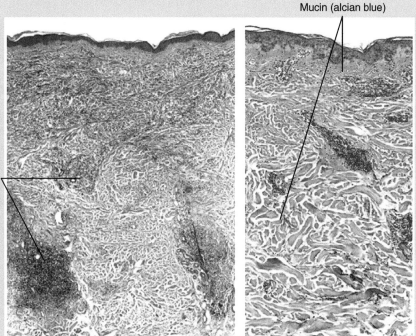

Mucin (alcian blue)

Dense nodular lymphocytic infiltrate

Hi: Superficial and deep perivascular and periadnexal cuff-like lymphocytic infiltrates, interstitial mucin deposits in the dermis, lack of epidermal changes such as junctional vacuolar degeneration or hyperparakeratosis.

DERMIS

VARIANT: **LE profundus (lupus panniculitis)**

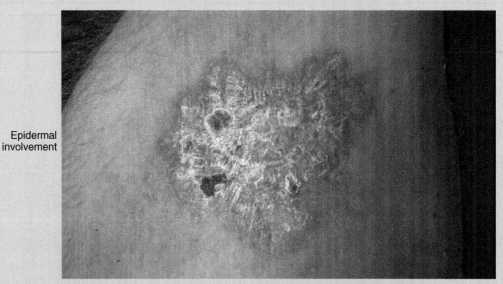

Epidermal involvement

Cl: Slightly elevated subcutaneous nodular lesion. The overlying epidermis is normal or retracted and sometimes may show involvement with erythema and firm hyperkeratosis. Ulcerations may occur.

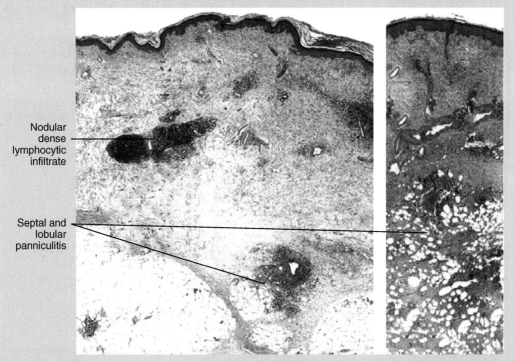

Nodular dense lymphocytic infiltrate

Septal and lobular panniculitis

Hi: Infiltrates in the deep dermis and in septae and lobules of the subcutaneous fat tissue. Conspicuous lack of neutrophils within the infiltrat. Admixture of plasma cells may be present.

DIFFERENTIAL DIAGNOSIS: Pernio (chilblains)

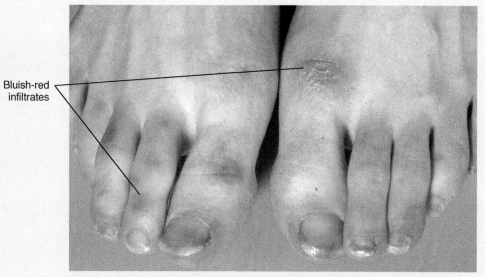

Bluish-red infiltrates

Cl: Blue-red edematous nodular swelling or infiltrates in acral localizations (fingers or toes), frequently associated with hyperhidrosis and acrocyanosis.

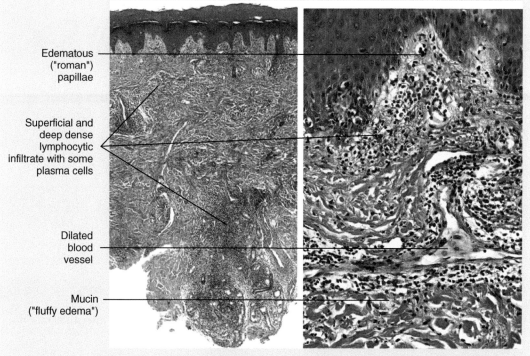

Edematous ("roman") papillae

Superficial and deep dense lymphocytic infiltrate with some plasma cells

Dilated blood vessel

Mucin ("fluffy edema")

Hi: Similar histological findings, but less prominent junctional vacuolization. Lymphocytes in edematous vessel walls; plasma cells may be present.

DERMIS

DIFFERENTIAL DIAGNOSIS: Lymphocytic infiltration (Jessner-Kanof)

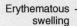

Erythematous swelling

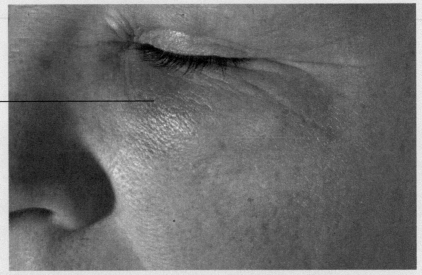

Cl: Circumscribed erythematous plaque-like swelling or infiltrate.

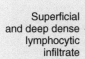

Superficial and deep dense lymphocytic infiltrate

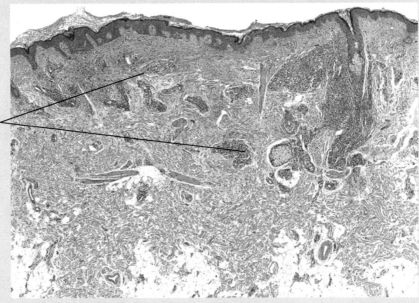

Hi: Perivascular lymphocytic infiltrates in all dermal layers. Sparse interstitial mucin deposits.

DIFFERENTIAL DIAGNOSIS: **Pseudolymphoma**

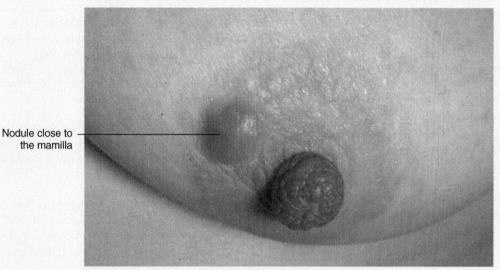

Nodule close to the mamilla

Cl: Usually solitary soft papule or nodule.

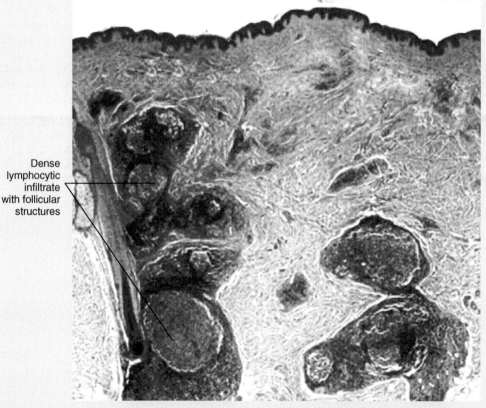

Dense lymphocytic infiltrate with follicular structures

Hi: Superficial and deep perivascular and interstitial lymphocytic infiltrates with admixture of plasma cells and eosinophils with or without follicular structures (lymphadenosis benigna cutis).

OTHER Diagnosis

Reticular erythematous mucinosis (REM syndrome) (*see* Chapter 7, Mucin, page 302): *Perivascular lymphocytic infiltrates in all dermal layers and sparse interstitial mucin deposits.*

Photoallergic and phototoxic reactions (*see* Chapter 2, Acute, pages 19, 83): *Apoptotic keratinocytes, spongiosis, perivascular infiltrate with eosinophils (especially in photoallergic reaction).*

Polymorphic light eruption (*see* Chapter 2, Acute, page 21): *Even though PLE is a monomorphous eruption in the affected individual, there are many (polymorphous) clinical features between individual patients, ranging from erythematous to papular or papulovesicular lesions, which appear exclusively in irradiated areas. Marked papillary dermal edema, blistering of the junctional zone, sleeve-like perivascular lymphocytic infiltrates with eosinophils. Epidermal changes with spongiosis may be present.*

References

Honigsmann, H. (2008). "Polymorphous light eruption." *Photodermatol Photoimmunol Photomed* **24**(3): 155–61.

Kuhn, A., M. Sonntag, P. Ruzicka, *et al.* (2003). "Histopathologic findings in lupus erythematosus tumidus: review of 80 patients." *J Am Acad Dermatol* **48**(6): 901–8.

Kuo, T. T., S. K. Lo, and H. L. Chan (1994). "Immunohistochemical analysis of dermal mononuclear cell infiltrates in cutaneous lupus erythematosus, polymorphous light eruption, lymphocytic infiltration of Jessner, and cutaneous lymphoid hyperplasia: a comparative differential study." *J Cutan Pathol* **21**(5): 430–6.

Molina-Ruiz, A. M., O. Sanmartin, C. Santonja, *et al.* (2013). "Spring and summer eruption of the elbows: a peculiar localized variant of polymorphous light eruption." *J Am Acad Dermatol* **68**(2): 306–12.

Naleway, A. L. (2002). "Polymorphous light eruption." *Int J Dermatol* **41**(7): 377–83.

Naleway, A. L., R. T. Greenlee, and J. W. Melski (2006). "Characteristics of diagnosed polymorphous light eruption." *Photodermatol Photoimmunol Photomed* **22**(4): 205–7.

Obermoser, G., R. D. Sontheimer, and B. Zelger (2010). "Overview of common, rare and atypical manifestations of cutaneous lupus erythematosus and histopathological correlates." *Lupus* **19**(9): 1050–70.

Pincus, L. B., P. E. LeBoit, D. S. Goddard, *et al.* (2010). "Marked papillary dermal edema – an unreliable discriminator between polymorphous light eruption and lupus erythematosus or dermatomyositis." *J Cutan Pathol* **37**(4): 416–25.

Rijlaarsdam, J. U., C. Nieboer, E. de Vries, and R. Willemze (1990). "Characterization of the dermal infiltrates in Jessner's lymphocytic infiltrate of the skin, polymorphous light eruption and cutaneous lupus erythematosus: differential diagnostic and pathogenetic aspects." *J Cutan Pathol* **17**(1): 2–8.

Vieira, V., J. Del Pozo, M. T. Yebra-Pimentel (2006). "Lupus erythematosus tumidus: a series of 26 cases." *Int J Dermatol* **45**(5): 512–17.

PROTOTYPE: Lymphomatoid papulosis (LYP), type A

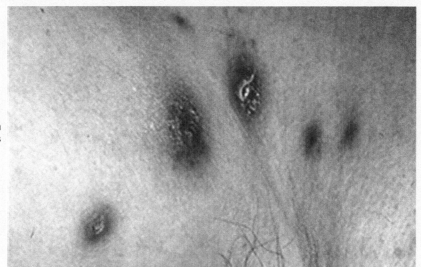

Papules with central necrosis

Cl: Disseminated or grouped recurrent, papulonecrotic lesions, which heal spontaneously within a few weeks, sometimes leaving behind varioliform scars.

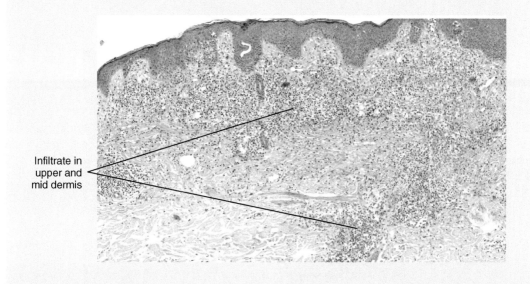

Infiltrate in upper and mid dermis

Lymphomatoid papulosis, type A

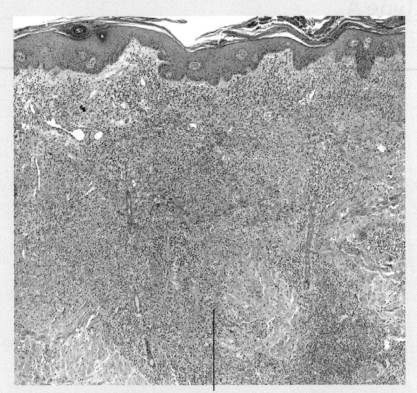

Lymphohistiocytic infiltrate with many eosinophils

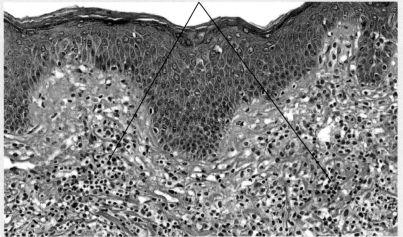

Infiltrate in
upper and
mid dermis

Hi: Various histological types (types A-E). Wedge shaped mixed infiltrate containing large atypical lymphocytes, small lymphocytes, histiocytes, neutrophils and eosinophils. Expression of CD30 by the large atypical lymphocytes (except in the MF-like type B), high mitotic activity, damage of blood vessel walls, ulceration, scar formation in regressing lesions.

Lymphomatoid papulosis, type A

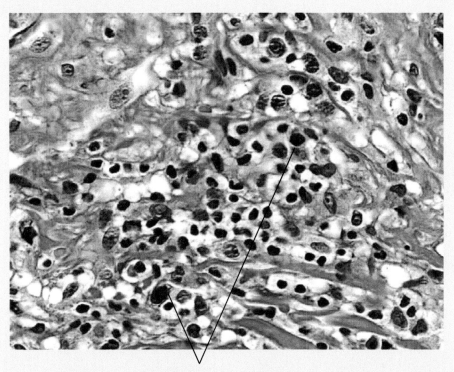

Atypical large CD30 positive lymphoid cells

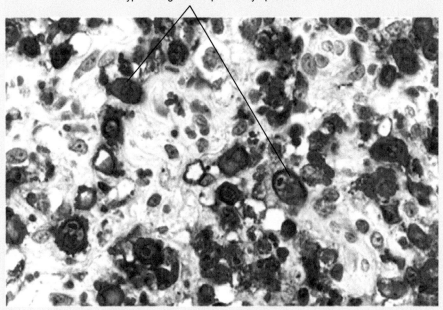

Hi: Scattered large CD30+ lymphocytes amongst an infiltrate with eosinophils and histiocytes.

VARIANTS: Types B, C, D, E, 6p25.3

Type B: Mycosis fungoides-like variant with epidermotropic small to medium-sized atypical lymphocytes with cerebriform nuclei and variable expression of CD30.

Type C: Cohesive sheets of large CD30+ lymphocytes with admixture of only a few inflammatory cells.

Type D: Epidermotropic infiltrate of small to medium-sized CD8+ and CD30+ atypical lymphocytes. Deeper perivascular infiltrates may be present.

Type E: Angiocentric and angiodestructive infiltrates of predominantly medium-sized atypical CD30+ and often CD8+ lymphocytes. Extensive hemorrhage, necrosis and ulceration.

6p25.3 translocation associated type: Pagetoid reticulosis-like epidermal involvement with usually prominent dermal nodule. Small to medium-sized atypical cells showing prominent periadnexal involvement. Frequent loss of T-cell markers (double negative for CD4 and CD8, however, beta F1+) with very high proliferative activity and diminished or lost expression of TIA-1. Positive FISH study with the 6p25.3 probe (the only subtype so far with reproducible genetic abnormality).

DIFFERENTIAL DIAGNOSIS

Primary cutaneous anaplastic large cell lymphoma (ALCL): Histological features identical to LyP type C with a nodular infiltrate of large CD30+ anaplastic lymphocytes. Expression of CD30 by more than 75% of large cells. Clinically solitary or grouped rapidly growing tumor.

Systemic anaplastic large cell lymphoma: Identical histological features to primary cutaneous ALCL and LyP type C, but often expression of ALK/p80 and EMA.

Mycosis fungoides (see Chapter 2, Psoriasiform and Chapter 3, Lichenoid, page 120): Patches and plaques are present. MF (patch/plaque) may histologically be indistinguishable from LyP type B and D, MF (transformation or tumor stage) may be similar to LyP C.

Primary cutaneous CD8+ aggressive epidermotropic cytotoxic T-cell lymphoma: Histologically similar to LyP type D, but no expression of CD30. Clinically rapidly evolving erosive and necrotic plaques and tumors.

Extranodal NK/T-cell lymphoma, nasal type and cutaneous gamma/delta lymphoma: Histologically similar to LyP type E, but clinically erosive and necrotic tumoral lesions, no spontaneous regression. Association with EBV in extranodal NK/T-cell lymphoma.

Lymphomatoid drug eruption: Variable features (Mycosis fungoides-like, Pseudolymphoma-like, Lupus erythematosus like, lichenoid, vasculitis-like).

Lymphomatoid contact dermatitis: Spongiosis, superficial and dense lymphoid infiltrate, eosinophils.

Hypersensitivity reaction (arthropod, scabies, infestations): Wedge-shaped infiltrate, mixed cellularity activated small to medium-sized lymphocytes, some of them with expression of CD30, neutrophils, eosinophils, plasma cells occasionally present, epidermal alterations).

References

Burg, G., G. Hoffmann-Fezer, *et al.* (1981). "Lymphomatoid papulosis: a cutaneous T-cell pseudolymphoma." *Acta Derm Venereol* **61**(6): 491–6.

Cardoso, J., P. Duhra, et al. (2012). "Lymphomatoid papulosis type D: a newly described variant easily confused with cutaneous aggressive CD8-positive cytotoxic T-cell lymphoma." *Am J Dermatopathol* **34**(7): 762–5.

El Shabrawi-Caelen, L., H. Kerl, *et al.* (2004). "Lymphomatoid papulosis: reappraisal of clinicopathologic presentation and classification into subtypes A, B, and C." *Arch Dermatol* **140**(4): 441–7.

Jokinen, C. H., G. M. Wolgamot, *et al.* (2007). "Lymphomatoid papulosis with CD1a+ dendritic cell hyperplasia, mimicking Langerhans cell histiocytosis." *J Cutan Pathol* **34**(7): 584–7.

Karai, L. J., M. E. Kadin, *et al.* (2013). "Chromosomal rearrangements of 6p25.3 define a new subtype of lymphomatoid papulosis." *Am J Surg Pathol* **37**(8): 1173–81.

DERMIS

Kempf, W. (2006). "CD30+ lymphoproliferative disorders: histopathology, differential diagnosis, new variants, and simulators." *J Cutan Pathol* **33 Suppl 1**: 58–70.

Kempf, W., D. V. Kazakov, *et al.* (2013). "Follicular lymphomatoid papulosis revisited: A study of 11 cases, with new histopathological findings." *J Am Acad Dermatol* **68**(5): 809–16.

Kempf, W., D. V. Kazakov, *et al.* (2013). "Angioinvasive lymphomatoid papulosis: a new variant simulating aggressive lymphomas." *Am J Surg Pathol* **37**(1): 1–13.

Macaulay, W. L. (1981). "Lymphomatoid papulosis. Thirteen years later." *Am J Dermatopathol* **3**(2): 165–7.

McQuitty, E., J. L. Curry, *et al.* (2014). "CD8-positive ("type D") lymphomatoid papulosis and its differential diagnosis." *J Cutan Pathol* **41**(2): 88–100.

Saggini, A., A. Gulia, *et al.* (2010). "A variant of lymphomatoid papulosis simulating primary cutaneous aggressive epidermotropic CD8+ cytotoxic T-cell lymphoma. Description of 9 cases." *Am J Surg Pathol* **34**(8): 1168–75.

Sharaf, M. A., P. Romanelli, *et al.* (2014). "Angioinvasive lymphomatoid papulosis: Another case of a newly described variant." *Am J Dermatopathol* **36**(3): e75–7.

Tomaszewski, M. M., G. P. Lupton, *et al.* (1995). "A comparison of clinical, morphological and immunohistochemical features of lymphomatoid papulosis and primary cutaneous CD30(Ki-1)-positive anaplastic large cell lymphoma." *J Cutan Pathol* **22**(4): 310–18.

DERMIS

PROTOTYPE: Acute febrile neutrophilic dermatosis (Sweet syndrome)

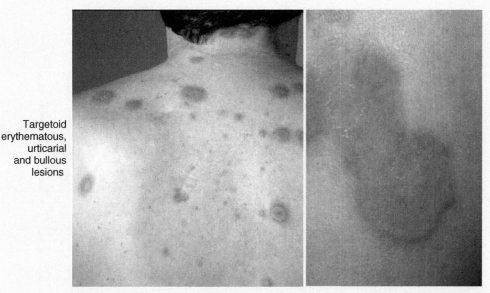

Targetoid erythematous, urticarial and bullous lesions

Cl: Succulent, tender, red juicy plaques or nodules, which eventually may get pustular, bullous and hemorrhagic. The patients present with fever and elevated neutrophil counts. Occasional association with myelomonocytic leukemia.

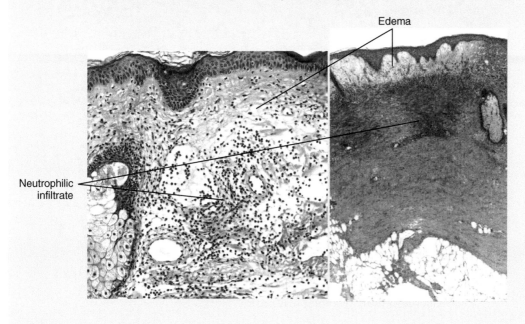

Edema

Neutrophilic infiltrate

Acute febrile neutrophilic dermatosis (Sweet syndrome)

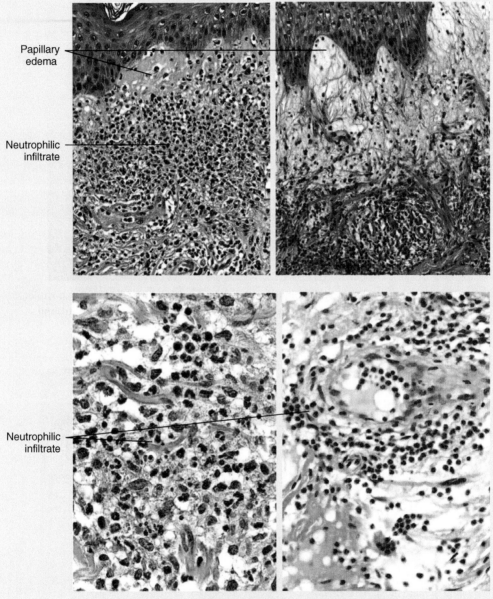

Papillary edema

Neutrophilic infiltrate

Neutrophilic infiltrate

Hi: Diffuse neutrophilic infiltrate extending to the deep dermis, marked papillary edema, leukocytoklasia with nuclear dust, no signs of vasculitis. Subcutaneous (panniculitis-like) Sweet syndrome may occur.

PROTOTYPE: Eosinophilic cellulitis (Wells syndrome)

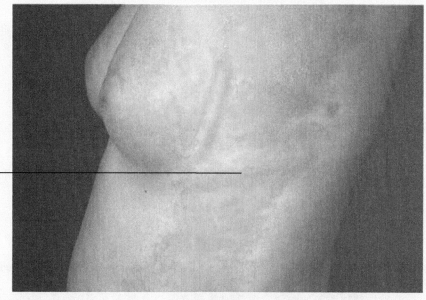

Erysipelas-like
and urticarial
lesions

Cl: Multiple circumscribed erythematous or urticarial lesions during the acute phase, which lasts a few days. In exceptional cases, large "geographical" erythemas, imitating erysipelas. Pruritic erythematous infiltrated lesions are typical for the late granulomatous stage.

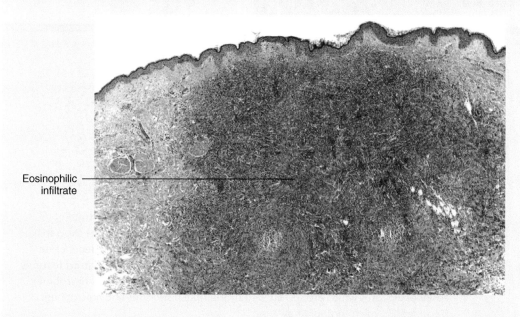

Eosinophilic
infiltrate

Eosinophilic cellulitis (Wells syndrome)

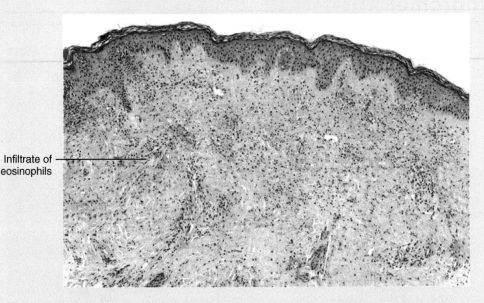

Infiltrate of eosinophils

Eosinophilic degeneration of collagen («flame figures») with eosinophils and eosinophilic dust

Eosinophils and nuclear dust

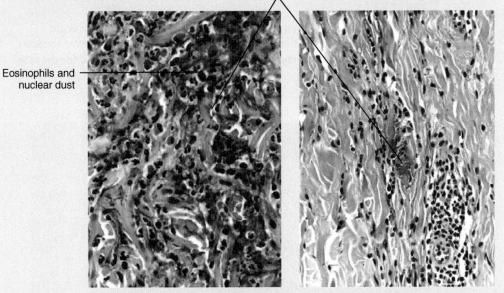

Hi: In the entire dermis, dense perivascular and diffuse interstitial infiltrate composed of eosinophilic granulocytes and few lymphocytes; edema of the papillary dermis; multiple eosinophilic flame figures consisting of eosinophilic degenerate collagenous cores surrounded by eosinophilic granulocytes; granulomatous features in late stages with eosinophilic micro-granulomas consisting of central necrobiotic eosinophilic cores which are surrounded by multiple histiocytes and macrophages ("eosinophilic micro-granulomas").

VARIANTS:

Early stage, with edematous urticarial infiltrate consisting mostly of eosinophilic granulocytes and few lymphocytes, rarely resembling erysipelas or classic urticaria.

Late stage, granulomatous infiltrations with multiple prominent eosinophilic micro-granulomas.

DERMIS

DIFFERENTIAL DIAGNOSIS: **Erysipelas**

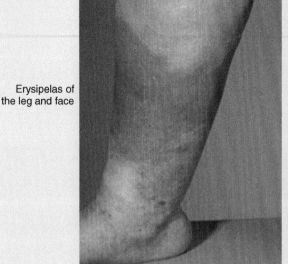 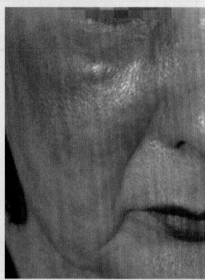

Erysipelas of the leg and face

Cl: There is a broad spectrum ranging from erythematous to hemorrhagic and bullous. The most typical presentation is a painful swelling and erythema with the tendency to centrifugal spread; due to mostly streptococcal infection of superficial lymph vessels. Preferential localizations are the legs and the face.

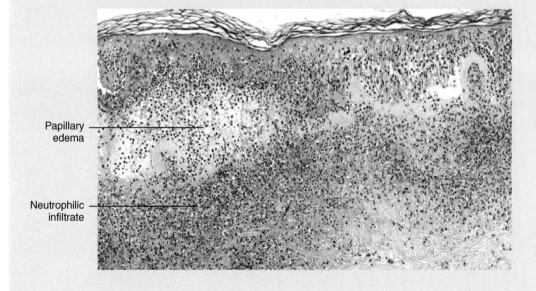

Papillary edema

Neutrophilic infiltrate

Erysipelas

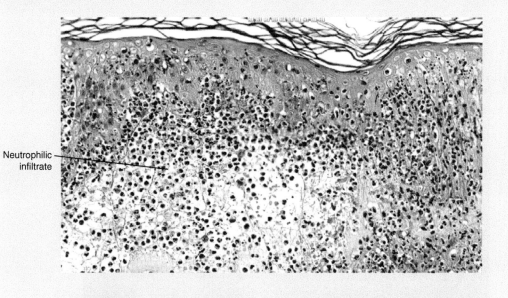

Neutrophilic infiltrate

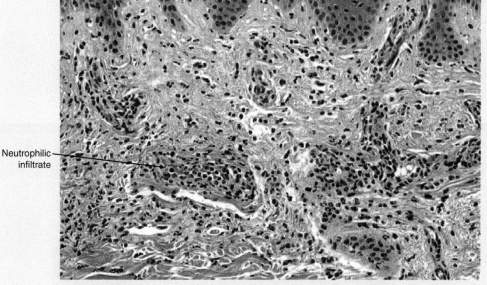

Neutrophilic infiltrate

Hi: Edema in the upper dermis, dilatation of vessels, neutrophilic infiltrate of variable density.

DERMIS

DIFFERENTIAL DIAGNOSIS: Abscess

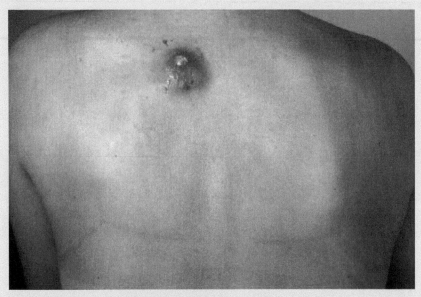

Cl: Circumscribed swelling with pustular core.

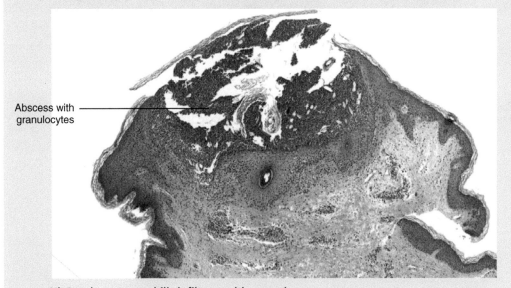

Abscess with granulocytes

Hi: Purulent neutrophilic infiltrate with necrosis.

DIFFERENTIAL DIAGNOSIS: Churg-Strauss syndrome (eosinophilic granulomatosis with polyangiitis)

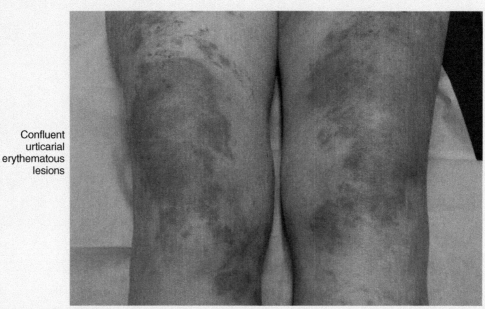

Confluent urticarial erythematous lesions

Cl: Purpuric erythema.

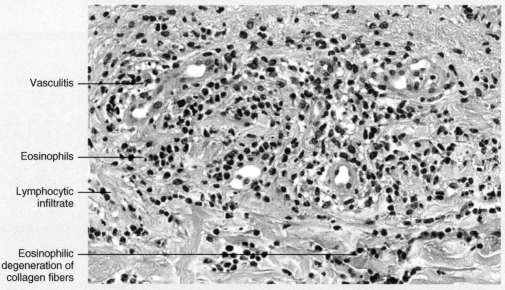

Vasculitis

Eosinophils

Lymphocytic infiltrate

Eosinophilic degeneration of collagen fibers

Hi: Eosinophilic vasculitis in conjunction with eosinophilic flame figures and/or eosinophilic palisading micro-granulomas. Eosinophilic vasculitis is paramount for the diagnosis.

DERMIS

DIFFERENTIAL DIAGNOSIS: **Bullous pemphigoid**

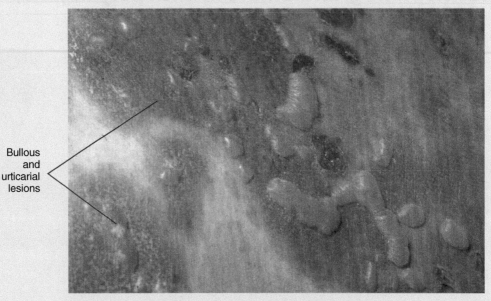

Bullous
and
urticarial
lesions

Cl: Erythema and tense bullae, occasionally hemorrhagic.

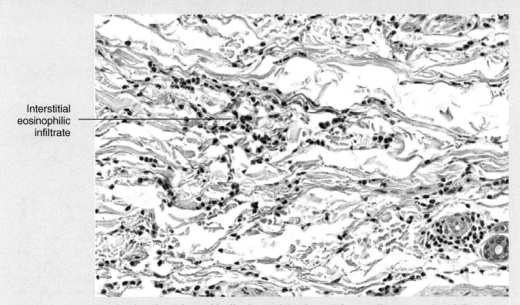

Interstitial
eosinophilic
infiltrate

Hi: Classic subepidermal bulla, in conjunction with an adjacent eosinophilic
infiltrate, occasionally studded with eosinophilic flame figures.

DIFFERENTIAL DIAGNOSIS: Pyoderma gangraenosum

Ulceration with elevated violaceous border

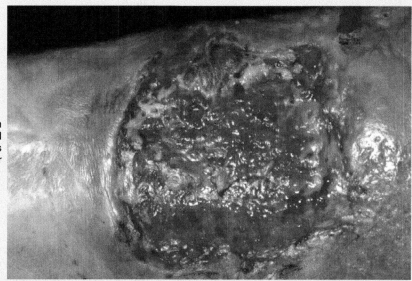

Cl: Centrifugally expanding ulcer with elevated undermined violaceous border.

Ulcer

Mixed inflammatory infiltrate

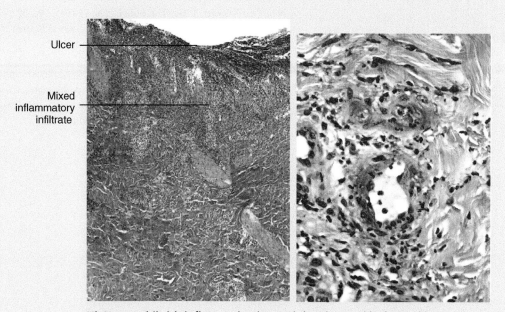

Hi: Neutrophil-rich inflammation beyond the ulcer and leukocytoklastic vasculitis with damaged vessel walls, intramural granulocytes, fibrin- and erythrocyte-extravasation.

Other Diagnosis

Arthropod bite reaction (*see* Chapter 3, Subepidermal blistering, page 129): *Circumscribed, wedge-shaped infiltrate, occasionally with flame figures.*

Eosinophilic folliculitis (HIV): Folliculitis with eosinophilic granulocytes, often spilling over into the adjacent dermis.

Eosinophilic fasciitis (Shulman syndrome) (*see* Sclerosis page 210): *Superficial and deep infiltrate, extending into the subcutis. Often sparse eosinophilic infiltrate in upper parts of the dermis, and dense infiltrate in the subcutis. Flame figures are not a constant feature.*

Comments

Classic "red" flame figures consist of a degenerate collagenous core surrounded by densely packed eosinophilic granulocytes and karyorrhexis. This type of flame figure may be encountered in all variants of eosinophil-rich inflammatory infiltrates.

Classic "blue" flame figures ("Churg-Strauss granuloma") consist of a rather large, strongly basophilic central necrobiotic collagenous core surrounded by densely packed neutrophilic granulocytes. Basophilic flame figures are most often associated with LE, rheumatoid arthritis and similar autoimmune disorders.

References

Aberer, W., K. Konrad, *et al.* (1988). "Wells' syndrome is a distinctive disease entity and not a histologic diagnosis." *J Am Acad Dermatol* **18**(1 Pt 1): 105–14.

Battistella, M., E. Bourrat, *et al.* (2012). "Sweet-like reaction due to arthropod bites: a histopathologic pitfall." *Am J Dermatopathol* **34**(4): 442–5.

Bonamigo, R. R., F. Razera, *et al.* (2011). "Neutrophilic dermatoses: part I." *An Bras Dermatol* **86**(1): 11–25; quiz 26–7.

Chan, M. P., L. M. Duncan, *et al.* (2013). "Subcutaneous Sweet syndrome in the setting of myeloid disorders: a case series and review of the literature." *J Am Acad Dermatol* **68**(6): 1006–15.

Draft, K. S., E. B. Wiser, *et al.* (2005). "Dermatopathology update of "newer" dermatologic manifestations of systemic disease." *Adv Dermatol* **21**: 101–32.

Moossavi, M. and D. R. Mehregan (2003). "Wells' syndrome: a clinical and histopathologic review of seven cases." *Int J Dermatol* **42**(1): 62–7.

Ratzinger, G., W. Burgdorf, *et al.* (2007). "Acute febrile neutrophilic dermatosis: a histopathologic study of 31 cases with review of literature." *Am J Dermatopathol* **29**(2): 125–33.

Stern, J. B., H. J. Sobel, *et al.* (1984). "Wells' syndrome: is there collagen damage in the flame figures?" *J Cutan Pathol* **11**(6): 501–5.

Wood, C., A. C. Miller, *et al.* (1986). "Eosinophilic infiltration with flame figures. A distinctive tissue reaction seen in Wells' syndrome and other diseases." *Am J Dermatopathol* **8**(3): 186–93.

PROTOTYPE: **Sarcoidosis**

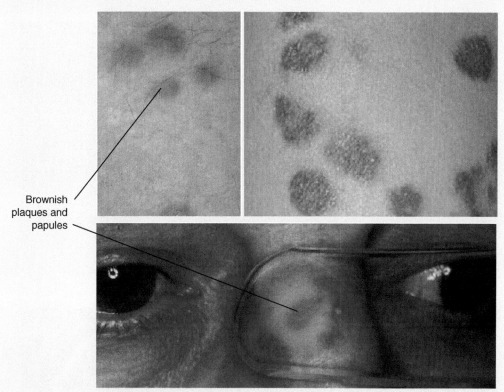

Brownish plaques and papules

Cl: There are many clinical forms of skin manifestations in sarcoidosis, which is basically a systemic disease with manifestations in various organs. Cutaneous lesions may appear as brown-bluish "sarcoid" erythemas, plaques, nodules, circinate lesions, subcutaneous infiltrates or cicatricial lesions.

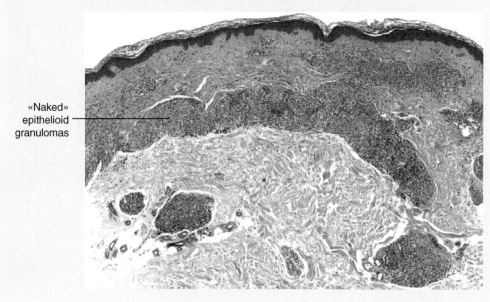

«Naked» epithelioid granulomas

Sarcoidosis

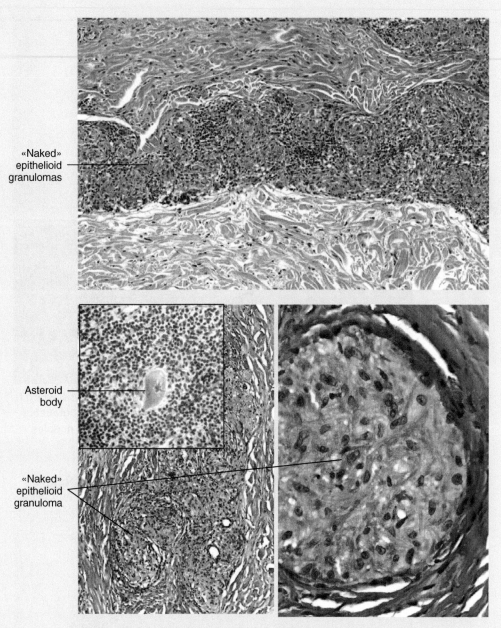

«Naked» epithelioid granulomas

Asteroid body

«Naked» epithelioid granuloma

Hi: Dermal nodular infiltrates of non-caseating "naked" (lacking an accompanying lymphocytic infiltrate) epithelioid granulomas; asteroid bodies in the cytoplasm of histiocytic giant cells. Admixture of only a few lymphocytes in most cases. Occasionally birefringent foreign body material is detectable by polarization (sarcoidal foreign body reaction).

VARIANT: **Granulomatosis disciformis (Miescher)**

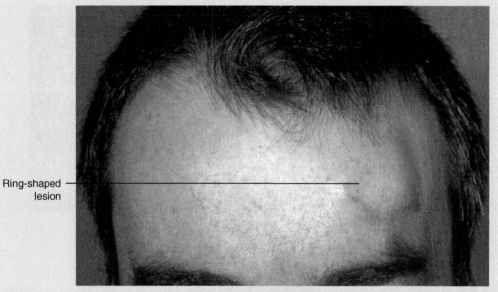

Ring-shaped
lesion

CI: Superficial disk-like or ring-shaped lesion, frequently on the forehead.

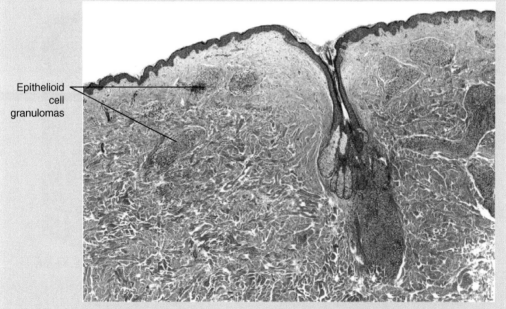

Epithelioid
cell
granulomas

Hi: "Naked" epithelioid cell granulomas in the upper dermis.

VARIANT: **Sarcoidosis (Lupus pernio)**

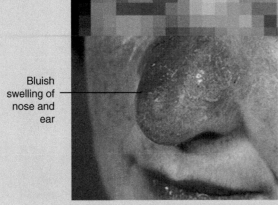
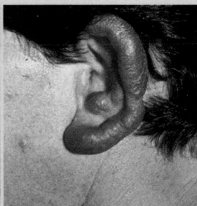

Bluish swelling of nose and ear

Cl: Bluish red infiltrated swelling, mostly in acral localization.

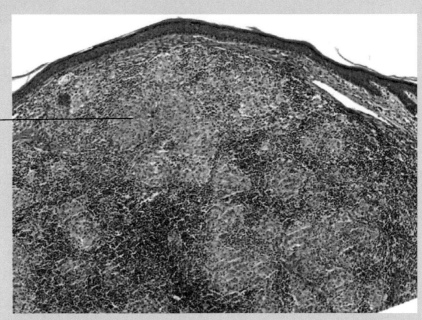

Epithelioid granulomas with admixture of numerous lymphocytes

Hi: Epithelioid granulomas accompanied by a dense lymphocytic infiltrate. Mostly located on the face, especially the nose.

Sarcoidosis associated syndromes

- *Löfgren-syndrome: Acute sarcoidosis, involvement of hilar lymph nodes, erythema nodosum, arthritis.*
- *Heerfordt –syndrome: Enlargement of parotis gland, uveitis, paresis of the facial nerve, fever.*
- *Ostitis cystica multiplex (Jüngling): Chronic fibrosing sarcoidosis, lupus pernio, bone cysts (distal phalanx of digits or toes).*

DIFFERENTIAL DIAGNOSIS: Cheilitis granulomatosa (Miescher)

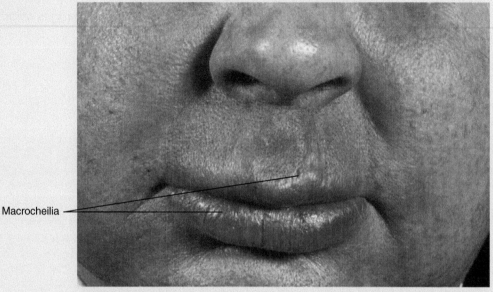

Macrocheilia

Cl: Lip swelling, may be associated with facial paresis and lingua plicata (Miescher-Melkersson-Rosenthal syndrome).

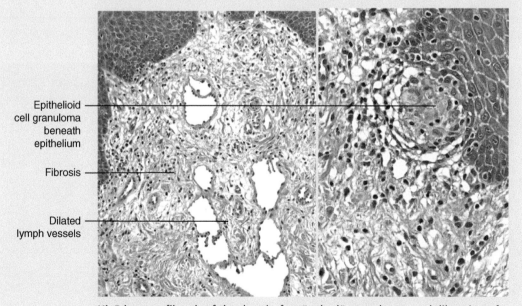

Epithelioid cell granuloma beneath epithelium

Fibrosis

Dilated lymph vessels

Hi: Edema or fibrosis of the dermis, few "naked" granulomas and dilatation of lymphatic vessels.

DIFFERENTIAL DIAGNOSIS: **Foreign body granuloma**

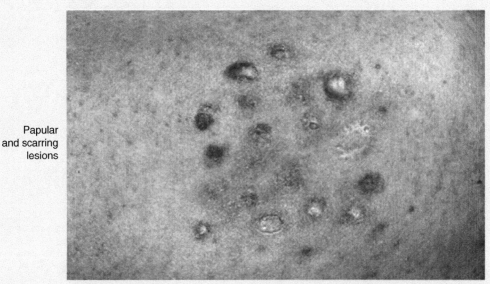

Papular
and scarring
lesions

Cl: Papules or scars.

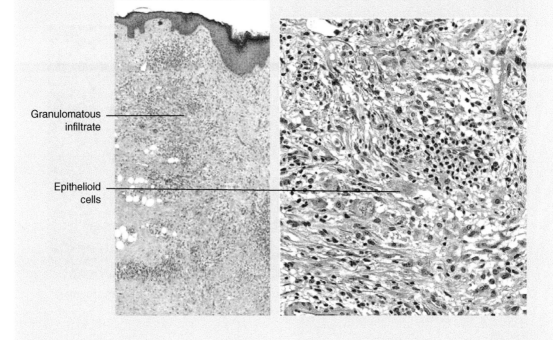

Granulomatous
infiltrate

Epithelioid
cells

Foreign body granuloma

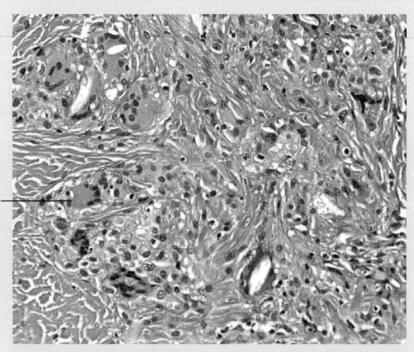

Langhans
type giant cells

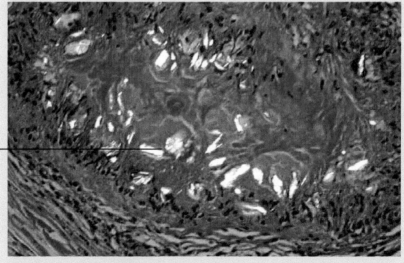

Birefringent
foreign bodies
within giant
cells (polarizing
light)

Hi: Detection of foreign bodies of various origin (filler substances, trauma-associated foreign material such as glass etc.).

DIFFERENTIAL DIAGNOSIS: Interstitial granulomatous dermatitis (with arthritis)

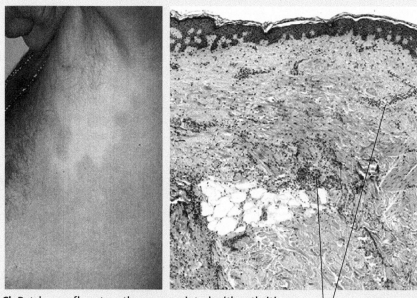

Distinct macular erythema on the left side of the thorax

Cl: Patchy confluent erythema associated with arthritis.

Interstitial and perivascular neutrophilic infiltrate

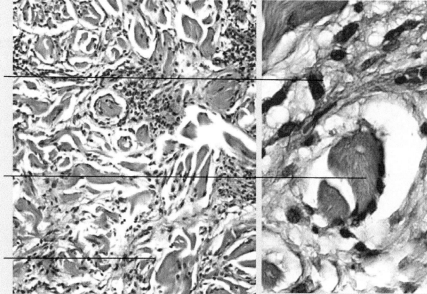

Histiocytes

«Free floating» collagen bundle surrounded by histiocytes

Interstitial histiocyte-rich infiltrate

Hi: Histiocyte-rich infiltrate, eosinophils, entrapment of collagen fibres, no necrobiosis. Typical "free floating" collagen bundles with peripheral rims of histiocytes.

Other Diagnosis

Granulomatous rosacea (*see* Chapter 8, Pilosebaceous unit, page 332): *Erythematous and slightly brownish plaques, papules or pustules in a centrofacial distribution involving the nose and cheeks. Histologically there is a folliculocentric granulomatous dermal infiltrate with epithelioid cells and multinucleated giant cells of the Langhans-type, telangiectasias in the upper dermis, lymphocytes, neutrophils and plasma cells, sebaceous hyperplasia*

Granuloma faciale (*see* Chapter 5, Localized, page 252): *violaceous brown-red infiltrated plaques, preferentially in the face of males. Histologically there is a lymphohistiocytic ("granulomatous") infiltrate with leukocytoklastic vasculitis. Many eosinophils and plasma cells are present.*

Granuloma annulare (*see* Dermis: Infiltrates: Granulomatous, with necrosis, page 187): *Necrobiotic areas containing mucin surrounded by a palisading histiocytic infiltrate or focal interstitial histiocyte-rich infiltrates (interstitial type).*

Crohn's disease: Non-caseating granulomas, clinical context crucial for diagnosis.

Mycobacterial infections (*see* Granulomatous, with necrosis, page 179): *Granulomas with or without necrosis (e.g. atypical mycobacteria) with admixture of neutrophils and lymphocytes. Detection of mycobacteria as acid-fast bacilli in Ziehl Neelsen stain, by PCR or tissue culture.*

Granulomatous cutaneous T-cell lymphoma (mycosis fungoides): Sarcoidal or granuloma annulare like pattern. Atypical small to medium-sized lymphocytes, epidermotropism in only half of the cases.

Erythema nodosum (*see* Chapter 6, Panniculitis, septal, page 268): *Multinucleated giant cells and mixed cellular infiltrate in the septa of the subcutaneous fat tissue. Erythema nodosum occurs together with lymphadenopathy and polyarthritis in the context of Loefgren syndrome in patients with acute sarcoidosis.*

Comment

The occurence of sarcoidal infiltrates due to foreign material in a preexisting scar may represent manifestation of systemic sarcoidosis and should be the starting point for further examinations.

References

Ball, N. J., G. T. Kho, *et al.* (2004). "The histologic spectrum of cutaneous sarcoidosis: a study of twenty-eight cases." *J Cutan Pathol* **31**(2): 160–8.

Brinster, N. K. (2008). "Dermatopathology for the surgical pathologist: a pattern-based approach to the diagnosis of inflammatory skin disorders (part II)." *Adv Anat Pathol* **15**(6): 350–69.

Haimovic, A., M. Sanchez, *et al.* (2012). "Sarcoidosis: a comprehensive review and update for the dermatologist: part I. Cutaneous disease." *J Am Acad Dermatol* **66**(5): 699 e1–18; quiz 717–18.

Mangas, C., M. T. Fernandez-Figueras, *et al.* (2006). "Clinical spectrum and histological analysis of 32 cases of specific cutaneous sarcoidosis." *J Cutan Pathol* **33**(12): 772–7.

Miida, H. and M. Ito (2010). "Tuberculoid granulomas in cutaneous sarcoidosis: a study of 49 cases." *J Cutan Pathol* **37**(4): 504–6.

Sanchez, J. L., A. C. Berlingeri-Ramos, et al. (2008). "Granulomatous rosacea." *Am J Dermatopathol* **30**(1): 6–9.

Tchernev, G., J. W. Patterson, *et al.* (2010). "Sarcoidosis of the skin – a dermatological puzzle: important differential diagnostic aspects and guidelines for clinical and histopathological recognition." *J Eur Acad Dermatol Venereol* **24**(2): 125–37.

Tomasini, C. and M. Pippione (2002). "Interstitial granulomatous dermatitis with plaques." *J Am Acad Dermatol* **46**(6): 892–9.

PROTOTYPE: **Lupus vulgaris**

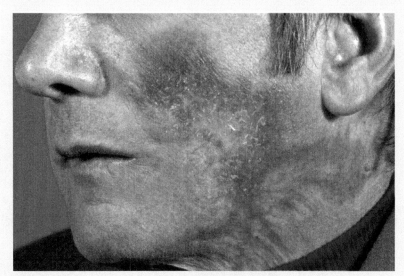

Atrophic
slightly scaling
red-brown
plaque with
scarring

Cl: Small nodules or atrophic, mutilating plaques. Verrucous variants with hyperkeratosis.

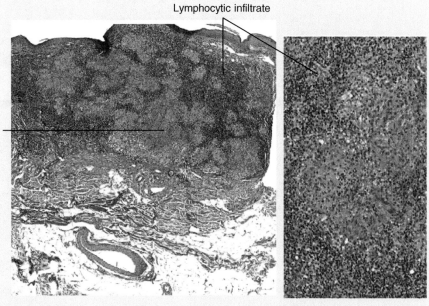

Lymphocytic infiltrate

Epithelioid
cell granulomas
with central
caseation

DERMIS

Lupus vulgaris

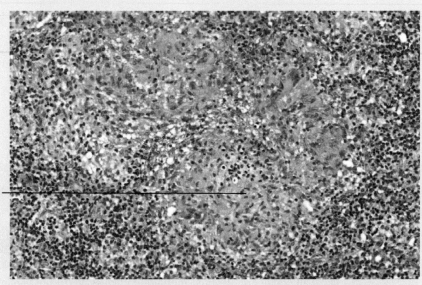

Epithelioid
cell granuloma
with lymphocytes

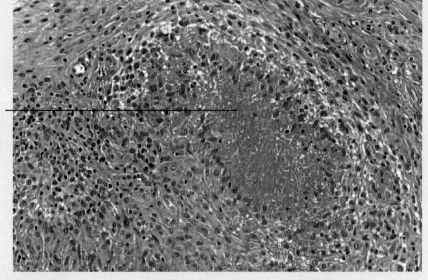

Epithelioid
cell granuloma
with central
necrosis

Hi: Small nodular dermal granulomas composed of pale histiocytes, few multinucleated Langhans cells, and a dense outer lymphocytic mantle. Central caseating necrosis may not always be present.

VARIANT: Atypical mycobacteriosis

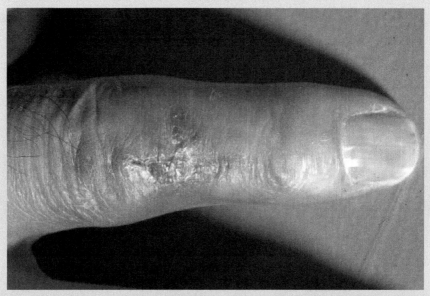

Hyperkeratotic lesion

DERMIS

Cl: Brown-bluish, mostly solitary nodular or plaque-like infiltrate with superficial ulceration and crust formation. Preferentially acral localization (hand or finger).

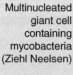

Multinucleated giant cell containing mycobacteria (Ziehl Neelsen)

Neutrophil-rich histiocytic infiltrates and granulomas

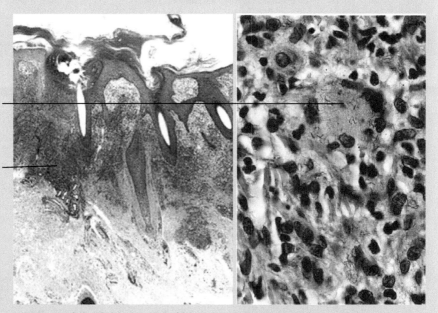

Hi: Neutrophil-rich histiocytic infiltrates and granulomas. Suppurative granulomas. Classic palisading pattern with caseation necrosis often missing. Detection of mycobacteria in some cases.

DERMIS

VARIANT: Papulonecrotic tuberculid

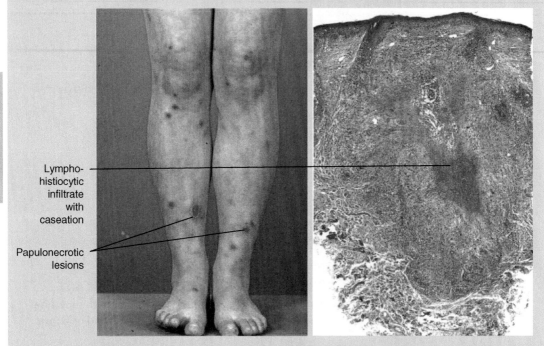

Lympho-
histiocytic
infiltrate
with
caseation

Papulonecrotic
lesions

Cl: Papulo-necrotic lesions, mostly in acral localization.

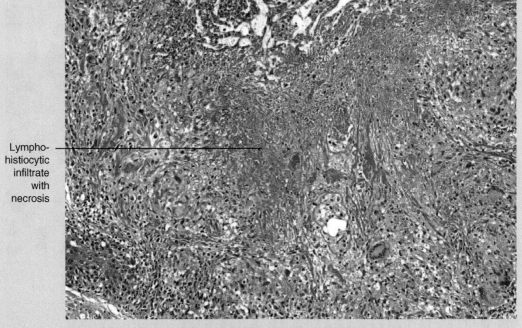

Lympho-
histiocytic
infiltrate
with
necrosis

Hi: Nodular or lymphohistiocytic infiltrates with or without caseation.
Small granulomas.

VARIANT: **Erythema induratum (Bazin)**

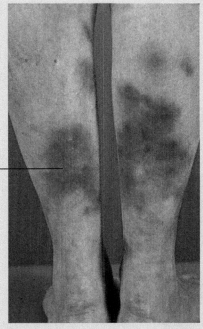

Contusiform lesions on the calfs

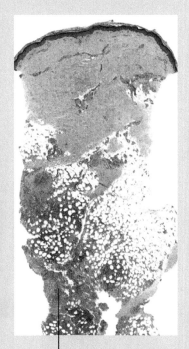

Cl: Contusiform plaques on the calfs, no ulceration.

Lymphohistiocytic infiltrate in the deep dermis and subcutis

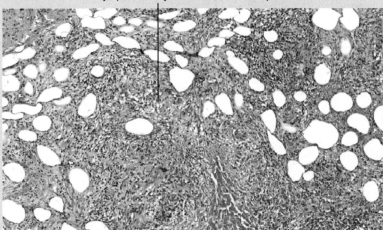

Hi: Suppurative granulomas. Mostly lobular panniculitis with or without accompanying vasculitis. Must be destinguished from nodal vasculitis and deep thrombophlebitis. Molecular detection of mycobacterial DNA in rare cases.

DERMIS

VARIANT: Lupus miliaris disseminatus faciei

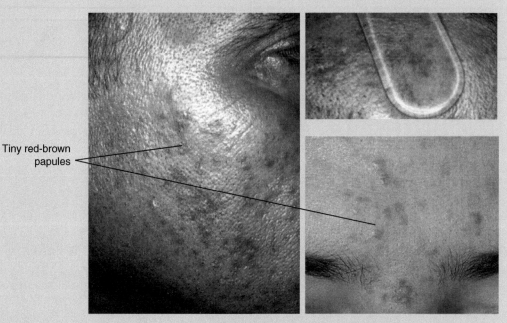

Tiny red-brown papules

Cl: Tiny red-brown papules, simulating acne.

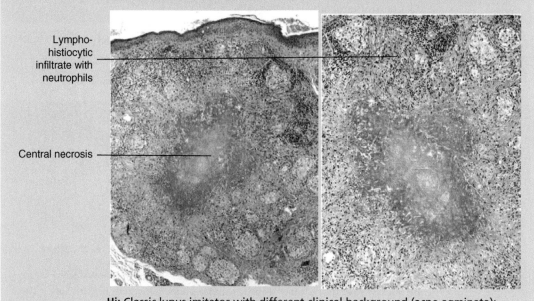

Lympho-histiocytic infiltrate with neutrophils

Central necrosis

Hi: Classic lupus imitator with different clinical background (acne agminata): marked central necrobiosis surrounded by lymphocytes and predominating histiocytes. No infectious organisms.

Tuberculosis cutis verrucosa: association of caseating granulomas with overlying verrucous epidermis.

DIFFERENTIAL DIAGNOSIS: Leishmaniasis

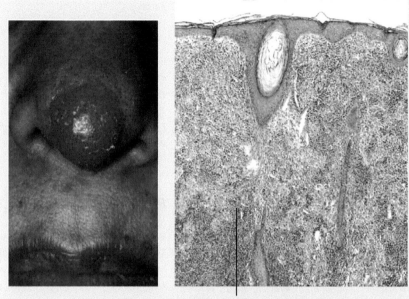

Lympho-histiocytic infiltrate with granulomatous features hugging the epidermis.

Cl: Cutaneous form shows a nodular infiltrate with tendency to ulceration.

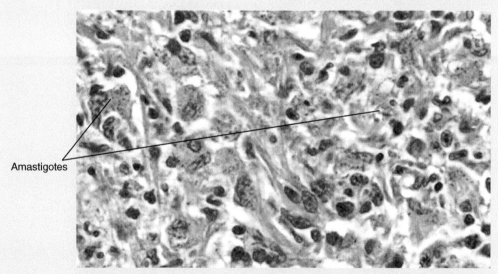

Amastigotes

Hi: Pale lymphohistiocytic infiltrate, with amastigotes. Plasma cells are typical.

DERMIS

Other Diagnosis

Granuloma annulare (*see* page 187): *Firm small skin-colored papules arranged in rings or arcs with predilection of the extensor aspects of extremities (especially fingers and backs of hands); in disseminated variant trunk is also involved. Less frequently hard, movable subcutaneous nodules are found. No pruritus.* Histology shows palisading granuloma, epitheloid cells, histiocytes, necrobiosis (degeneration of collagen), with deposits of mucin.

Sarcoidosis (*see* Granulomatous, without necrosis, page 169): *"Naked granulomas" with subtle or absence of a peripheral lymphocytic mantle. Slight central necrobiosis may be present in exceptional cases. No mycobacteria detectable.*

Necrobiosis lipoidica: Yellow plaques and patches, frequently on the shins of women, erythematous border, central atrophy. Ulceration may occur. Histologically layers of confluent necrobiosis are seen throughout the dermis, alternating with layers of palisading lymphohistiocytic granulomatous infiltrate with multinucleated giant cells, plasma cells are common.

Rheumatoid nodules: Eosinophilic necrobiotic areas surrounded by palisading histiocytic infiltrate.

Elastolytic giant cell granuloma: Solitary or annular and confluent lesions, preferentially in light exposed areas. Histology shows annular granulomas with central necrobiosis, simulating granuloma annulare and many giant cells containing inclusions of phagocytized fibers.

Foreign body granuloma (*see* Granulomatous, with necrosis, page 175): *Look for birefringent foreign body particles.*

Granulomatous acne/rosacea (*see* Chapter 8, Pilosebaceous unit, page 332): *Perifollicular infiltrates. No necrobiotic caseating centers amidst granulomas. No typical palisading pattern.*

Granuloma faciale (*see* Chapter 5, Localized, page 252): *Brownish plaques, frequently in the face or on the forehead. Lymphohistiocytic, granulomatous infiltrate with eosinophils and plasma cells with signs of leukocytoklastic small vessel vasculitis.*

References

Farina, M. C., M. I. Gegundez, *et al.* (1995). "Cutaneous tuberculosis: a clinical, histopathologic, and bacteriologic study." *J Am Acad Dermatol* **33**(3): 433–40.

Min, K. W., J. Y. Ko, *et al.* (2012). "Histopathological spectrum of cutaneous tuberculosis and non-tuberculous mycobacterial infections." *J Cutan Pathol* **39**(6): 582–95.

PROTOTYPE: **Granuloma annulare**

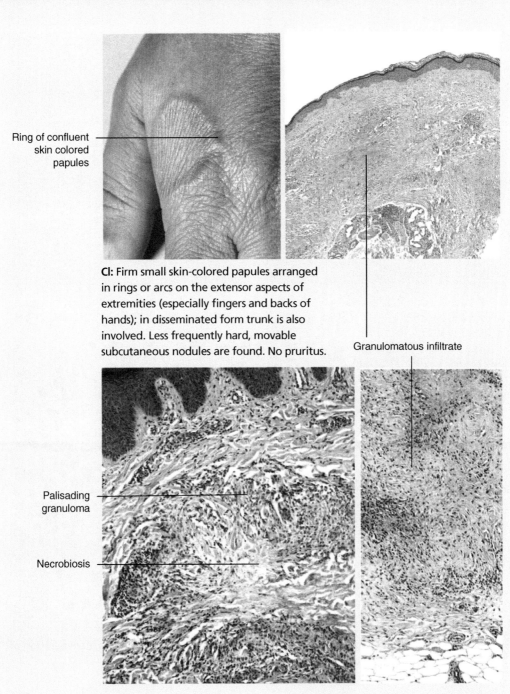

Ring of confluent skin colored papules

Cl: Firm small skin-colored papules arranged in rings or arcs on the extensor aspects of extremities (especially fingers and backs of hands); in disseminated form trunk is also involved. Less frequently hard, movable subcutaneous nodules are found. No pruritus.

Granulomatous infiltrate

Palisading granuloma

Necrobiosis

DERMIS

Granuloma annulare

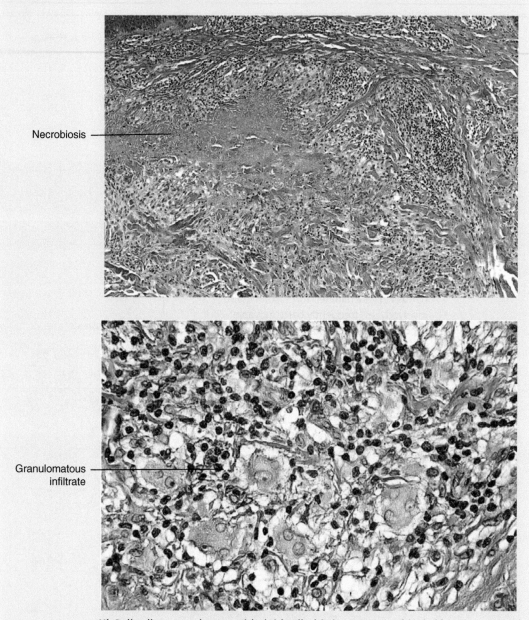

Necrobiosis

Granulomatous infiltrate

Hi: Palisading granuloma, epitheloid cells, histiocytes, necrobiosis (degeneration of collagen), deposits of mucin, a few eosinophils.

DERMIS

VARIANT: **Deep granuloma annulare**

Interstitial form: no necrobiosis, interstitial histiocyte-rich infiltrate

Perforating granuloma annulare

Subcutaneous granuloma annulare

Granuloma annulare in scars (zoster)

DERMIS

DERMIS

VARIANT: **Annular elastolytic giant cell granuloma**

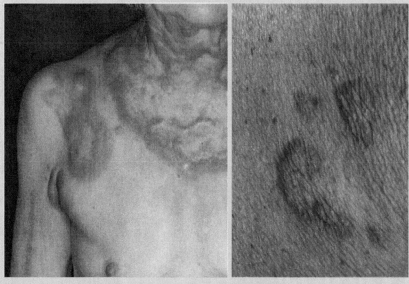

Confluent anular lesions with elevated border and central atrophy

Cl: Annular or plaque-like lesions with elevated borders.

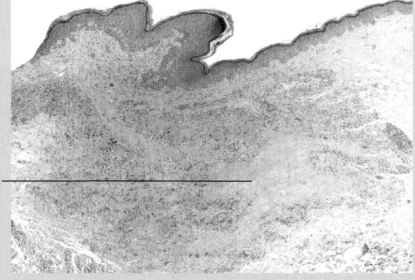

Palisading histiocyte-rich infiltrate with central necrobiosis

Comment

May be identical with necrobiotic xanthogranuloma (*see* DEPOSITION AND STORAGE, Lipids, page 295).

Annular elastolytic giant cell granuloma

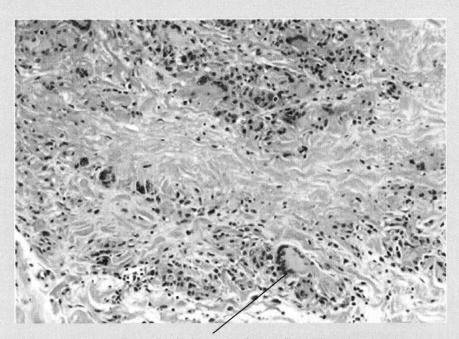

Giant cells with fragments of elastic fibers (elastophagocytosis)

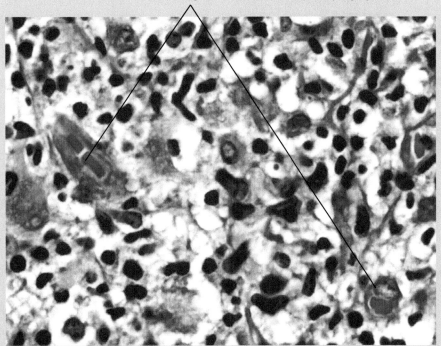

Hi: Palisading granuloma with central necrosis; multinucleated giant cells with inclusions of fibrous material in the periphery.

DERMIS

DERMIS

DIFFERENTIAL DIAGNOSIS: **Necrobiosis lipoidica**

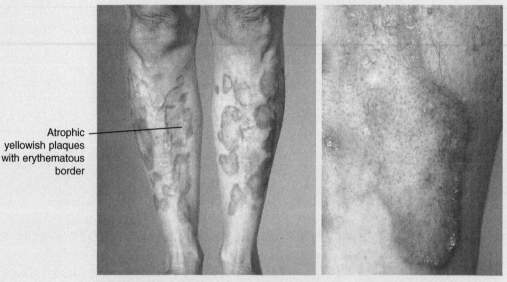

Atrophic yellowish plaques with erythematous border

Cl: Brownish and yellowish atrophic plaques with erythematous border, preferentially on the lower extremities; frequent association with diabetes mellitus.

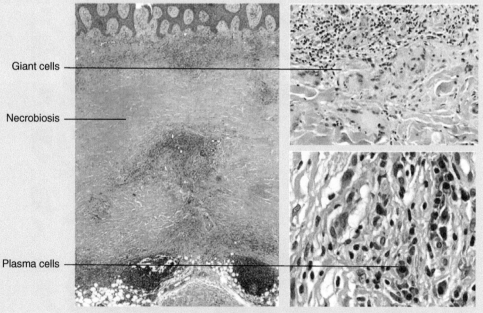

Giant cells

Necrobiosis

Plasma cells

Hi: Alternating horizontal layers of degenerated collagen and granulomatous infiltrate throughout all levels of the dermis.

DIFFERENTIAL DIAGNOSIS: **Rheumatoid nodule**

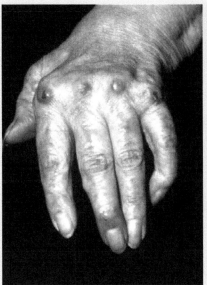 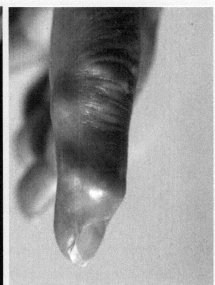

CI: Hard nodules, preferentially on elbows, fingers, feet and knees, in conjunction with rheumatoid arthritis.

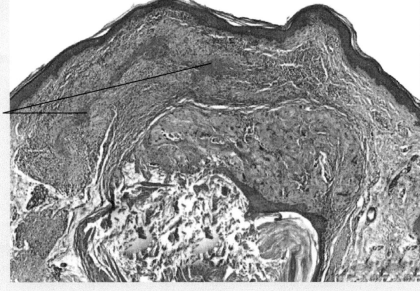

Necrobiosis

DERMIS

Rheumatoid nodule

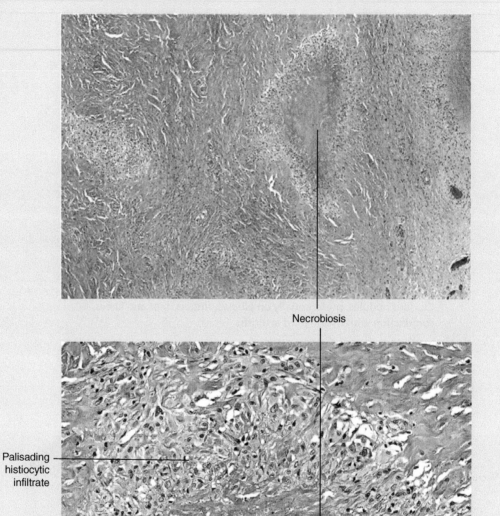

Necrobiosis

Palisading
histiocytic
infiltrate

Hi: Area of eosinophilic degeneration of collagenous and fibrous tissue, surrounded by a palisaded granulomatous infiltrate. Vasculitis is exceptionally rare.

References

Al-Hoqail, I. A., A. M. Al-Ghamdi, *et al.* (2002). "Actinic granuloma is a unique and distinct entity: a comparative study with granuloma annulare." *Am J Dermatopathol* **24**(3): 209–12.

Bardach, H. G. (1977). "Granuloma annulare with transfollicular perforation." *J Cutan Pathol* **4**(2): 99–104.

Bergman, R., Z. Pam, *et al.* (1993). "Localized granuloma annulare. Histopathological and direct immunofluorescence study of early lesions, and the adjacent normal-looking skin of actively spreading lesions." *Am J Dermatopathol* **15**(6): 544–8.

Cota, C., G. Ferrara, *et al.* (2012). "Granuloma annulare with prominent lymphoid infiltrates ("pseudolymphomatous" granuloma annulare)." *Am J Dermatopathol* **34**(3): 259–62.

Friedman-Birnbaum, R., S. Weltfriend, *et al.* (1989). "A comparative histopathologic study of generalized and localized granuloma annulare." *Am J Dermatopathol* **11**(2): 144–8.

Guitart, J., A. Zemtsov, *et al.* (1991). "Diffuse dermal histiocytosis. A variant of generalized granuloma annulare." *Am J Dermatopathol* **13**(2): 174–8.

Gunes, P., F. Goktay, *et al.* (2009). "Collagen-elastic tissue changes and vascular involvement in granuloma annulare: a review of 35 cases." *J Cutan Pathol* **36**(8): 838–44.

Limas, C. (2004). "The spectrum of primary cutaneous elastolytic granulomas and their distinction from granuloma annulare: a clinicopathological analysis." *Histopathology* **44**(3): 277–82.

Patterson, J. W. (1988). "Rheumatoid nodule and subcutaneous granuloma annulare. A comparative histologic study." *Am J Dermatopathol* **10**(1): 1–8.

DERMIS

PROTOTYPE: **Granulomatous mycosis fungoides**

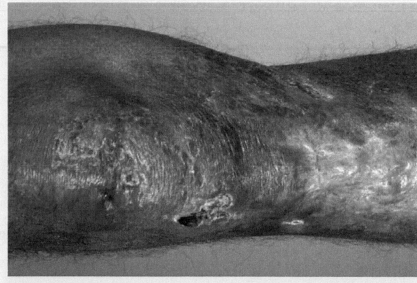

Brownish
plaques

Cl: Patches and plaques.

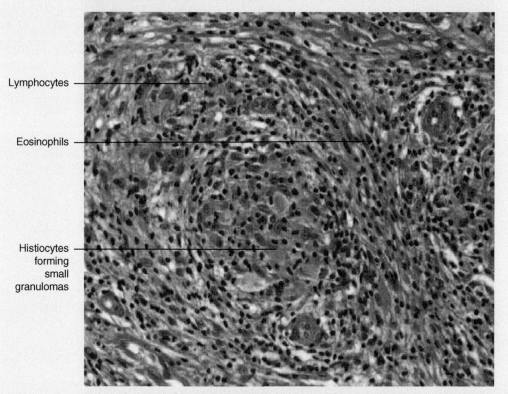

Lymphocytes

Eosinophils

Histiocytes
forming
small
granulomas

Hi: Lymphocytic infiltrate with prominent accumulations of histiocytes macrophages
and giant cells. Epidermotropism in half of the cases only.

VARIANT: **Granulomatous slack skin**

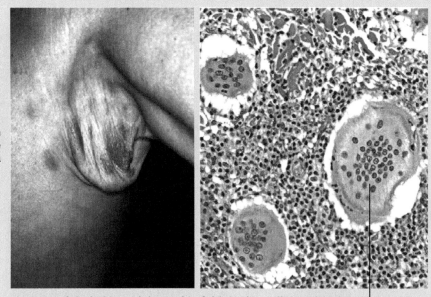

Pendulous skin
fold in the
axilla

Cl: Areas of slack skin with large skin folds in the axillae and groins.

Scattered large multinucleated giant cells with emperipolesis

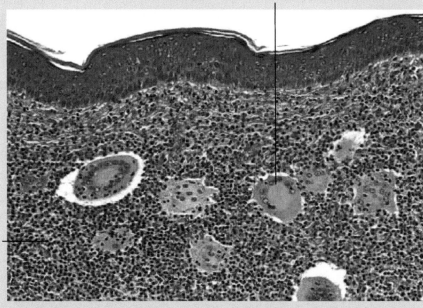

Lymphocytic
infiltrate

Hi: Disseminated large multinucleated giant cells with emperipolesis "floating" within the tumorous lymphocytic infiltrate.

DERMIS

DERMIS

DIFFERENTIAL DIAGNOSIS: Langerhans cell histiocytosis (Histiocytosis X)

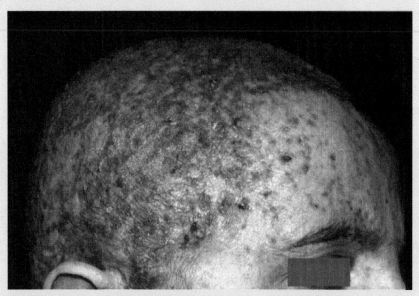

Scaly crusty lesions in a child

Cl: Letterer-Siwe: children, scaly and crusty lesions on the head and at diaper and seborrheic sites. Hand-Schüller-Christian: adults, intertriginous areas. Additional symptoms present in both forms.

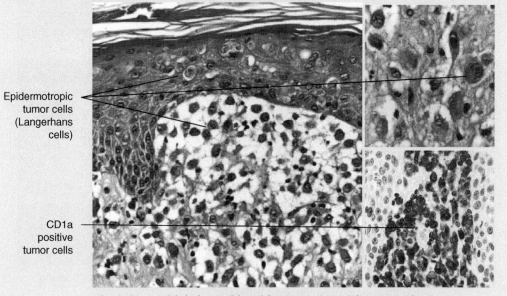

Epidermotropic tumor cells (Langerhans cells)

CD1a positive tumor cells

Hi: Histiocyte-rich lesions with epidermotropic proliferations of cells with large, pale, vesicular nucleus and abundant slightly eosinophilic or amphophilic cytoplasm (Langerhans cells).

DIFFERENTIAL DIAGNOSIS: Non-X-histiocytoses: Juvenile xanthogranuloma

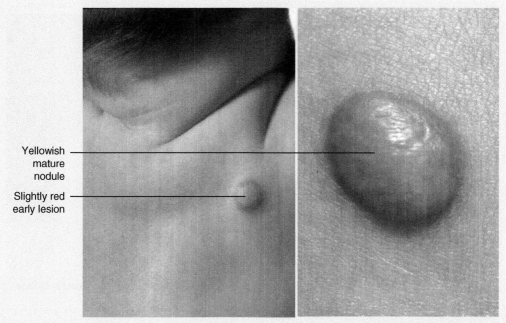

Yellowish mature nodule

Slightly red early lesion

Cl: Solitary or multiple papules.

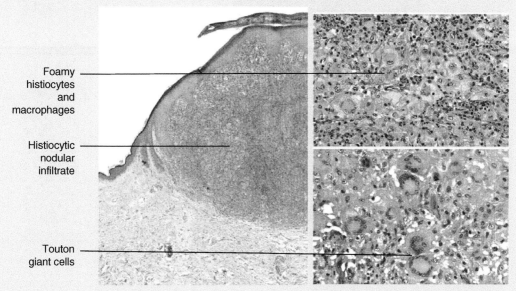

Foamy histiocytes and macrophages

Histiocytic nodular infiltrate

Touton giant cells

Hi: Histology shows a dense infiltrate of macrophages with abundant slightly eosinophilic cytoplasm in early lesions, whereas in mature lesions foamy cells and Touton giant-cells are seen.

DIFFERENTIAL DIAGNOSIS: Benign cephalic histiocytosis (close relationship to JXG)

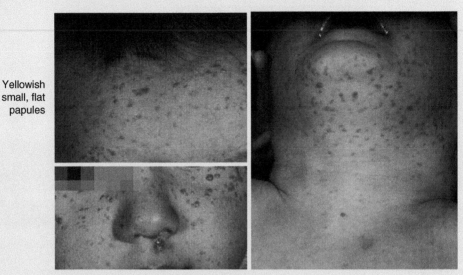

Yellowish small, flat papules

CI: Slightly raised, small red to yellowish papules, mostly in the head and face area of children.

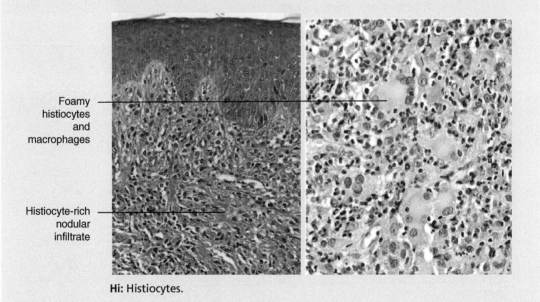

Foamy histiocytes and macrophages

Histiocyte-rich nodular infiltrate

Hi: Histiocytes.

DIFFERENTIAL DIAGNOSIS: Congenital self-healing reticulohistiocytosis (Hashimoto-Pritzker)

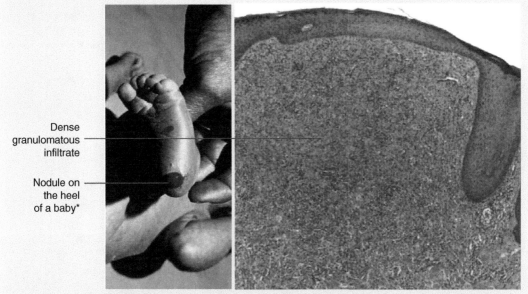

Dense granulomatous infiltrate

Nodule on the heel of a baby*

Cl: Congenital small solitary or multiple nodules. No systemic involvement. Spontaneous regression *(Bonifazi et al 1982)*.

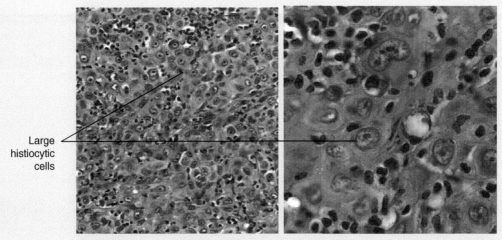

Large histiocytic cells

Hi: Large mono-or multinucleated cells with abundant eosinophilic or ground-glass like cytoplasm.

DERMIS

DIFFERENTIAL DIAGNOSIS: **Multicentric reticulohistiocytosis (MRH, lipoid dermatoarthritis)**

Multicentric reticulohistocytosis (MRH)

Multinucleated giant cell

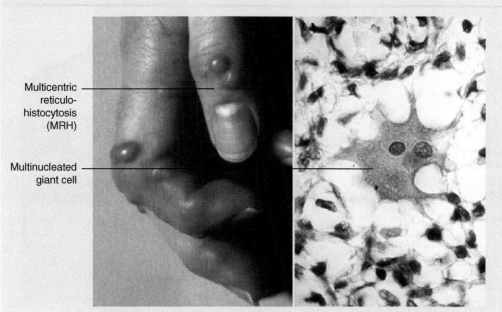

Cl: Systemic disease, predominantly in middle-aged women, showing multiple small firm nodules; may be paraneoplastic.
Hi: Histiocyte-rich infiltrates with PAS-positive multinucleated giant cells.

DIFFERENTIAL DIAGNOSIS: Progressive nodular histiocytosis (PNH)

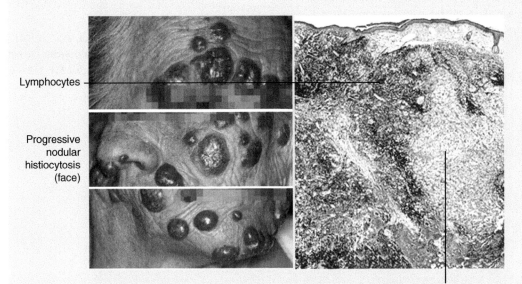

Lymphocytes

Progressive nodular histiocytosis (face)

Histiocytes in PNH

Cl: Progressive development of widespread nodular and tumorous lesions. Good general health, absence of systemic symptoms.

Hi: Massive infiltrate of histiocytes, intermixed with lymphocytes.

Other Diagnosis

Necrobiotic xanthogranuloma *(see* Chapter 7, Lipids, page 295)*: Mostly in association with IgG paraproteinemia. Yellowish indurated plaques. Histology reveals collagen degeneration, sheets of foamy cells, cholesterol clefts and Touton type giant cells.*

References

Bonifazi, E., R. Caputo, *et al.* (1982). "Congenital self-healing histiocytosis." *Arch Dermatol* **118**(4): 267–72.

Caputo, R. (1998). *Text-atlas of Histiocytic Syndromes.* London, Martin Dunitz.

Gianotti, F. and R. Caputo (1985). "Histiocytic syndromes: a review." *J Am Acad Dermatol* **13**(3): 383–404.

Schaumburg-Lever, G., E. Rechowicz, *et al.* (1994). "Congenital self-healing reticulohistiocytosis – a benign Langerhans cell disease." *J Cutan Pathol* **21**(1): 59–66.

PROTOTYPE: **Circumscribed scleroderma (morphea)**

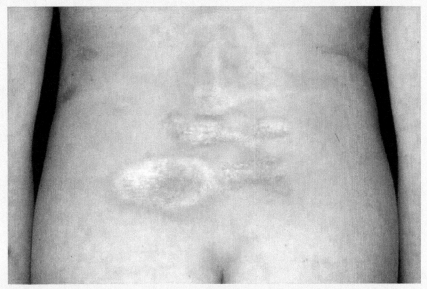

White-yellow
sclerotic
plaques
with lilac ring

CI: Centrifugally spreading erythema with progressive central white-yellow induration with loss of adnexal structures. Border often with purple tones (lilac ring) as sign of disease activity.

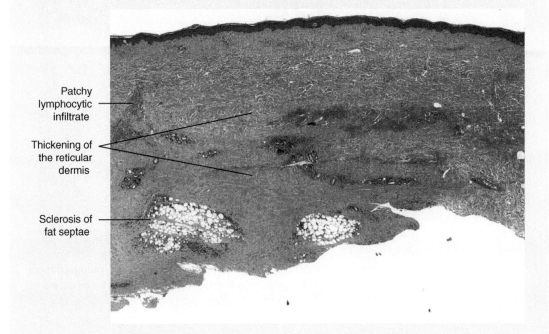

Patchy
lymphocytic
infiltrate

Thickening of
the reticular
dermis

Sclerosis of
fat septae

DERMIS

Circumscribed scleroderma (morphea)

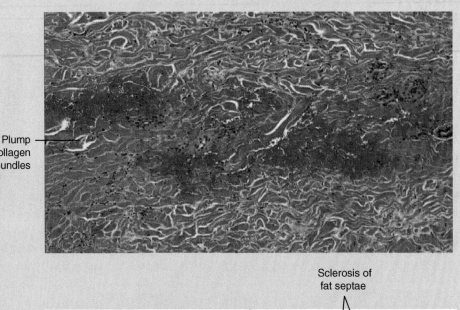

Plump collagen bundles

Sclerosis of fat septae

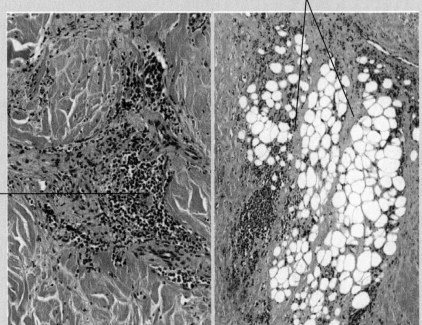

Scattered lymphocytic infiltrate

Hi: Epidermis normal or atrophic, thickening of the reticular dermis, plump collagen bundles, reduction of elastic fibres, sclerosis of fat septae, scattered lymphocytic infiltrate, occasionally plasma cells, nodular aggregation of lymphocytes at the dermal-subcutis border.

VARIANTS:

Early stage morphea: edema in the upper dermis, lymphocytic infiltrate, occasional plasma cells and eosinophils

Late stage morphea: prominent fibrosis and thickening of the reticular dermis, thickening of collagen bundles, dilatation of blood vessels, entrapping of sweat glands and adnexal structures in higher levels of the dermis and embedded in thickened collagen bundles.

Morphea profunda: fibrosis extending into the subcutaneous tissue. *Sclero-lichen:* combination of morphea and histological pattern of lichen sclerosus et atrophicus.

DERMIS

DIFFERENTIAL DIAGNOSIS: Systemic scleroderma

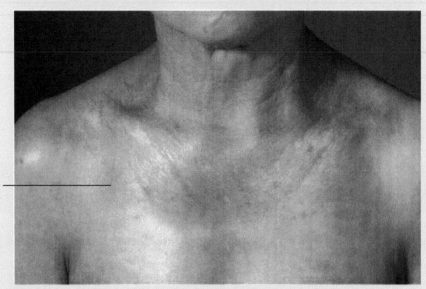

Tight
sclerotic
skin

Cl: Systemic disorder with potential involvement of internal structures and variable presentation on the skin, which is hardened and thickened; acral forms and generalized forms. Raynaud phenomenon.

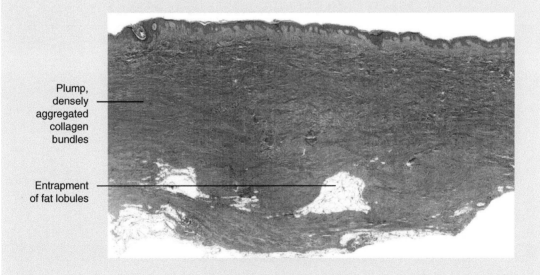

Plump,
densely
aggregated
collagen
bundles

Entrapment
of fat lobules

Systemic scleroderma

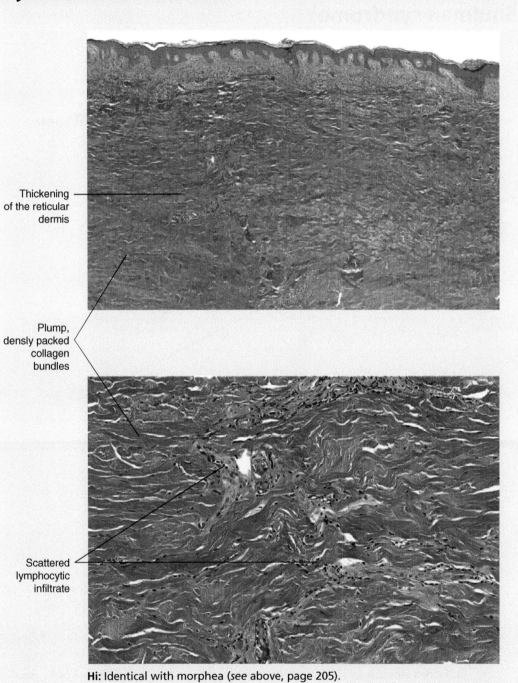

Thickening of the reticular dermis

Plump, densly packed collagen bundles

Scattered lymphocytic infiltrate

Hi: Identical with morphea (*see* above, page 205).

DERMIS

DIFFERENTIAL DIAGNOSIS: Eosinophilic fasciitis (Shulman syndrome)

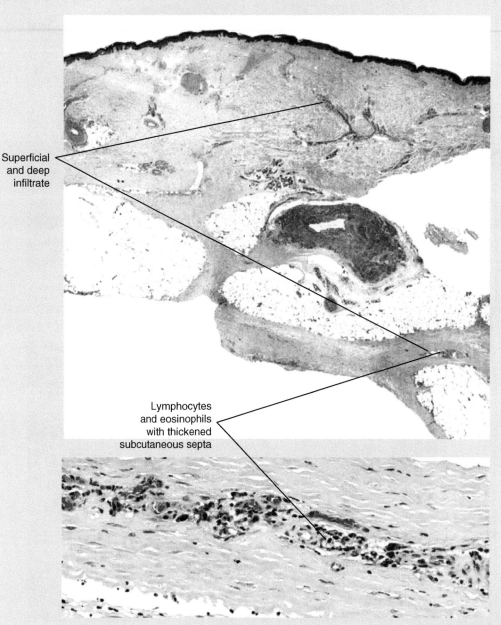

Superficial and deep infiltrate

Lymphocytes and eosinophils with thickened subcutaneous septa

Cl: Sudden symmetrical hardening of skin, preferentially in young adults, lack of Raynaud phenomenon.
Hi: Deep morphea pattern, involving subcutaneous septa.

Eosinophilic fasciitis (Shulman syndrome)

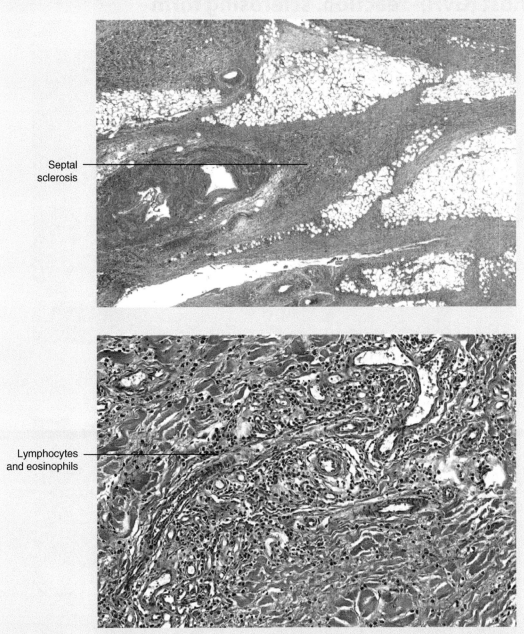

Septal
sclerosis

Lymphocytes
and eosinophils

Hi: In addition to sclerosis of the dermis and fat septa, there is conspicuous sclerosis
of fascia. Tissue eosinophilia may be present.

DERMIS

DIFFERENTIAL DIAGNOSIS: Chronic graft-versus-host (GvH)- reaction, sclerosing form

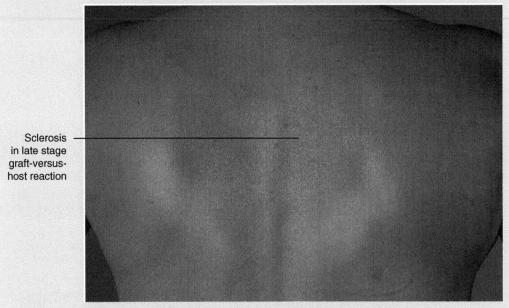

Sclerosis in late stage graft-versus-host reaction

Cl: Hardening of the skin, similar to systemic sclerosis.

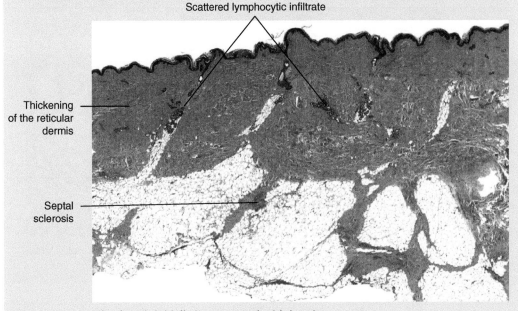

Scattered lymphocytic infiltrate

Thickening of the reticular dermis

Septal sclerosis

Hi: Sclerosis initially in upper and mid dermis.

DIFFERENTIAL DIAGNOSIS: **Stasis dermatitis**

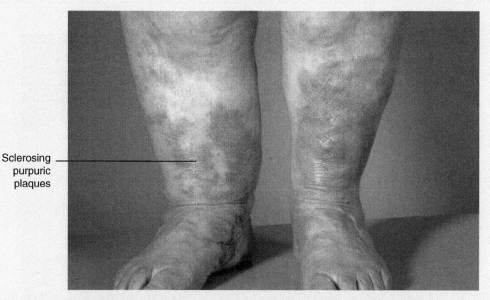

Sclerosing purpuric plaques

Cl: Pruritic eczematous skin changes with red to brown pigmentation, commonly in conjunction with chronic venous insufficiency and thus preferential localization on the lower legs.

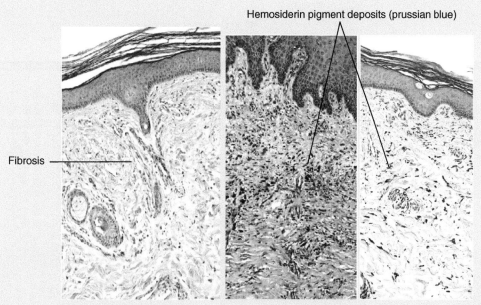

Hemosiderin pigment deposits (prussian blue)

Fibrosis

Hi: Acanthosis and variable degree of spongiosis, Erythrocyte extravasation, edema in the upper dermis, sclerosis in the mid and lower dermis may be present, hemosiderin deposits in all dermal layers.

DERMIS

DIFFERENTIAL DIAGNOSIS: Connective tissue nevus

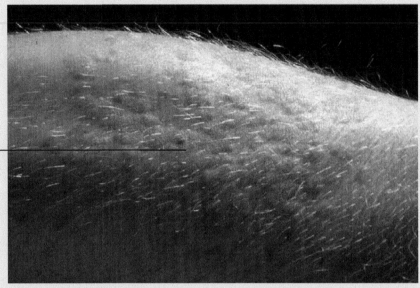

Flat confluent papules

Cl: Soft papules or plaque.

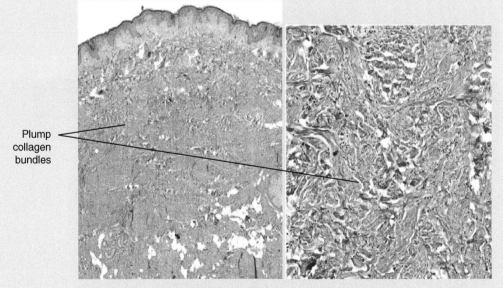

Plump collagen bundles

Hi: Thickened and disarranged collagen as well as elastic fibers. No infiltrate.

Other Diagnosis

Lipodermatosclerosis: Sclerosis and hemosiderin deposits in all dermal layers. Subtle infiltrate.

Nephrogenic fibrosing dermopathy: Increased number of (CD34+) fibroblasts, interstitial mucin deposits.

Scar: Loss of elastic fibres and adnexal structures.

References

Barzilai, A., A. Lyakhovitsky, *et al.* (2003). "Keloid-like scleroderma." *Am J Dermatopathol* **25**(4): 327–30.

Cowper, S. E. and R. Bucala (2003). "Nephrogenic fibrosing dermopathy: suspect identified, motive unclear." *Am J Dermatopathol* **25**(4): 358.

Dhaliwal, C. A., A. I. MacKenzie, *et al.* (2014). "Perineural inflammation in morphea (localized scleroderma): systematic characterization of a poorly recognized but potentially useful histopathological feature." *J Cutan Pathol* **41**(1): 28–35.

Elliott, C. J., J. P. Sloane, *et al.* (1987). "The histological diagnosis of cutaneous graft versus host disease: relationship of skin changes to marrow purging and other clinical variables." *Histopathology* **11**(2): 145–55.

Goh, C., A. Biswas, *et al.* (2012). "Alopecia with perineural lymphocytes: a clue to linear scleroderma en coup de sabre." *J Cutan Pathol* **39**(5): 518–20.

Grant, J. (1979). "Fasciitis and scleroderma." *Am J Dermatopathol* **1**(1): 89.

Kucher, C., X. Xu, *et al.* (2005). "Histopathologic comparison of nephrogenic fibrosing dermopathy and scleromyxedema." *J Cutan Pathol* **32**(7): 484–90.

Montes, L. F., S. Gay, *et al.* (1978). "Scleroderma." *J Cutan Pathol* **5**(3): 150–1.

Rahbari, H. (1989). "Histochemical differentiation of localized morphea-scleroderma and lichen sclerosus et atrophicus." *J Cutan Pathol* **16**(6): 342–7.

Satter, E. K., J. S. Metcalf, *et al.* (2006). "Can scleromyxedema be differentiated from nephrogenic fibrosing dermatopathy by the distribution of the infiltrate?" *J Cutan Pathol* **33**(11): 756–9.

Torres, J. E. and J. L. Sanchez (1998). "Histopathologic differentiation between localized and systemic scleroderma." *Am J Dermatopathol* **20**(3): 242–5.

Walling, H. W., M. D. Voigt, *et al.* (2004). "Lichenoid graft vs. host disease following liver transplantation." *J Cutan Pathol* **31**(2): 179–84.

Walters, R., M. Pulitzer, *et al.* (2009). "Elastic fiber pattern in scleroderma/morphea." *J Cutan Pathol* **36**(9): 952–7.

Wriston, C. C., A. I. Rubin, *et al.* (2008). "Nodular scleroderma: a report of 2 cases." *Am J Dermatopathol* **30**(4): 385–8.

PROTOTYPE: **Reactive perforating collagenosis**

Ulceration

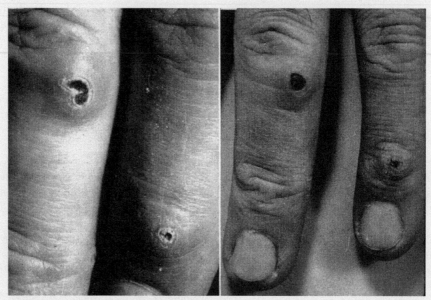

Cl: Pruritic papules with small ulcers with eschar.

Extrusion
of collagen

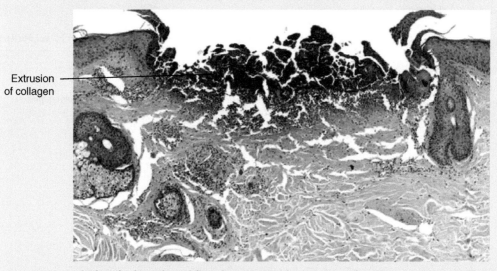

Hi: Sharply demarkated flat ulceration with extrusion of collagen and elastic fibers, covered by debris and neutrophils. Subtle infiltrate mainly of neutrophils in the upper dermis.

DERMIS

VARIANTS: **Elastosis perforans serpiginosa (perforating elastosis)**

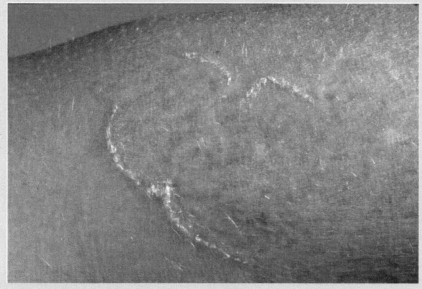

Upper extremity

Cl: Tiny keratotic papules forming annular lines.

Degenerated elastotic material and mixed cellular infiltrate

Hi: Increased number and sizes of elastic fibres in upper dermis; small transepithelial channel with extrusion of elastic fibers; degenerated elastotic material; mixed cellular infiltrate with neutrophils.

Hyperkeratosis follicularis et parafollicularis in cutem penetrans (Kyrle's disease): *Hyperkeratotic dome-shaped papules with a central plug, sometimes in a linear arrangement. Histology shows an intraepithelial channel; crater filled with parakeratotic horn.*

DIFFERENTIAL DIAGNOSIS: Keratosis pilaris

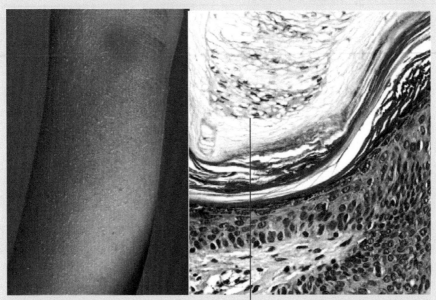

Cl: Tiny keratotic papules.

Hyperkeratosis in the hair follicular ostium

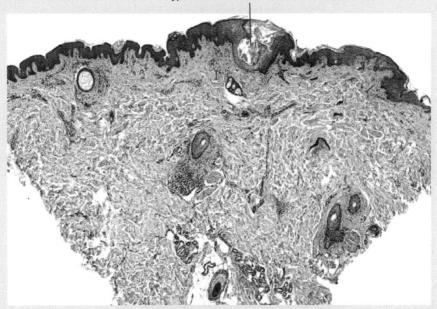

Hi: Hyperparakeratosis in the hair follicle ostia.

Comment

Reactive perforating collagenosis is considered as variant of prurigo with deep excoriation and subsequent extrusion of collagen and elastic fibers. It is often associated with diabetes mellitus and chronic hepatic or renal failure.

References

Beck, H. I., F. Brandrup, *et al.* (1988). "Adult, acquired reactive perforating collagenosis. Report of a case including ultrastructural findings." *J Cutan Pathol* **15**(2): 124–8.

Faver, I. R., M. S. Daoud, et al. (1994). "Acquired reactive perforating collagenosis. Report of six cases and review of the literature." *J Am Acad Dermatol* **30**(4): 575–80.

Golitz, L. (1985). "Follicular and perforating disorders." *J Cutan Pathol* **12**(3–4): 282–8.

Millard, P. R., E. Young, *et al.* (1986). "Reactive perforating collagenosis: light, ultrastructural and immunohistological studies." *Histopathology* **10**(10): 1047–56.

Yanagihara, M., T. Fujita, *et al.* (1996). "The pathogenesis of the transepithelial elimination of the collagen bundles in acquired reactive perforating collagenosis. A light and electron microscopical study." *J Cutan Pathol* **23**(5): 398–403.

CHAPTER 5
Vessels

Atlas of Dermatopathology: Practical Differential Diagnosis by Clinicopathologic Pattern, First Edition.
Edited by Günter Burg MD, Werner Kempf MD, and Heinz Kutzner MD. Co-Editors: Josef Feit MD, and Laszlo Karai MD.
© 2015 John Wiley & Sons, Ltd. Published 2015 by John Wiley & Sons, Ltd.

VESSELS

PROTOTYPE: **Purpura fulminans**

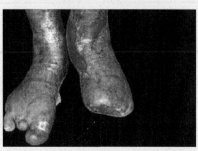

Mutilations following purpura fulminans

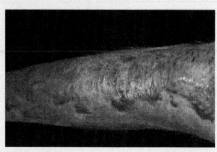

Cl: Purpura fulminans is a severe, life-threatening disorder caused by disseminated intravascular coagulation. Due to multiple causes, including meningococcal sepsis, intravascular coagulation leads to widespread cutaneous hemorrhage, preferentially on the extremities with ecchymoses, blistering and necrosis of various degree.

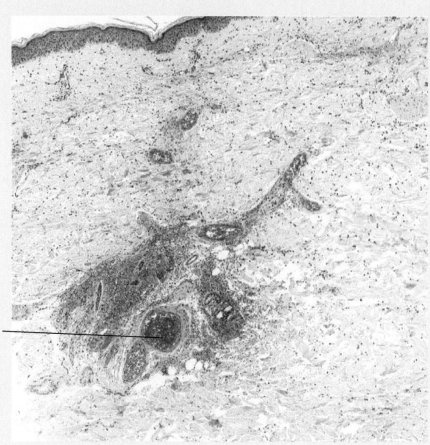

Intravascular occlusion and hemorrhage

Purpura fulminans

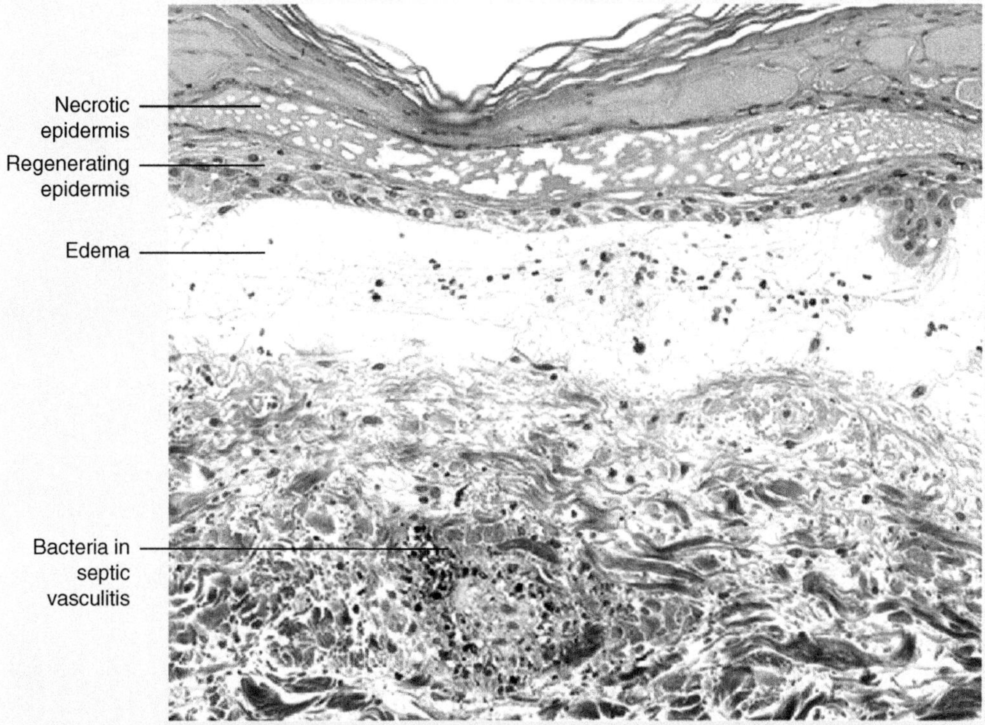

Necrotic
epidermis

Regenerating
epidermis

Edema

Bacteria in
septic
vasculitis

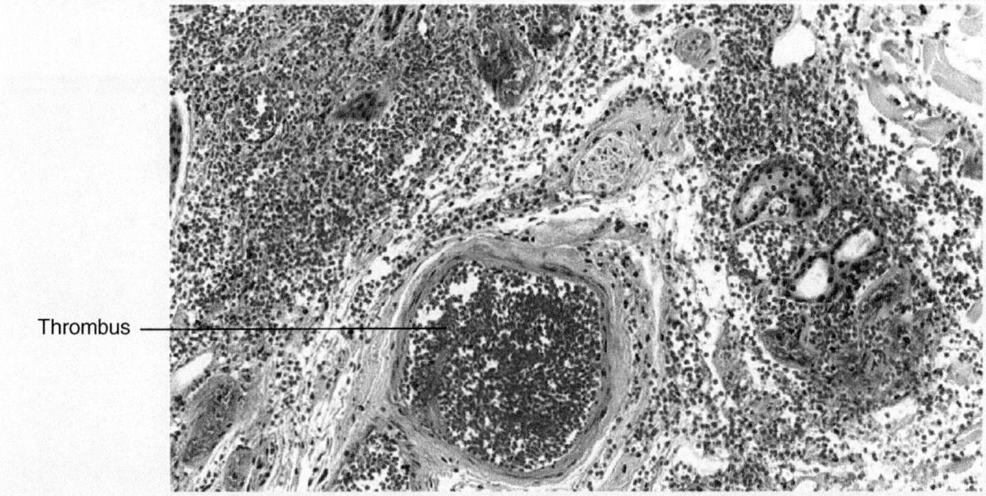

Thrombus

Hi: Occlusion of small vessels by fibrin thrombi, extensive extravasation of
erythrocytes, no or sparse inflammation, in advanced stages massive necrosis with
ulceration.

VESSELS

VARIANT: **Septic vasculitis**

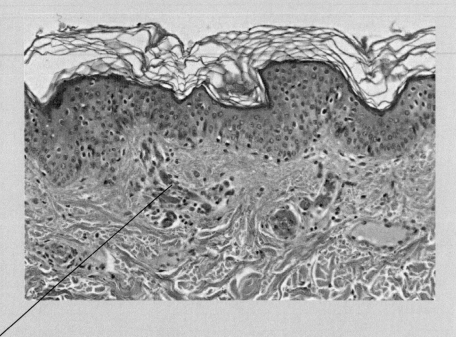

Intravascular
occlusion

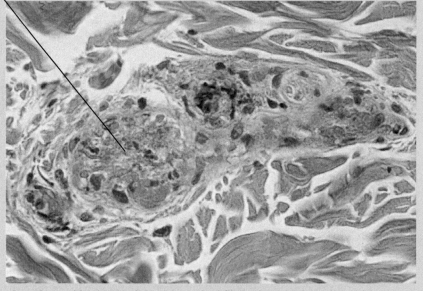

Hi: Leukocytoklastic vasculitis with marked fibrin thrombi, bacteria within the vessel lumen and vessel wall. Neutrophilic infiltrate and karyorrhexis often very discrete.

VARIANT: **Coumarin necrosis**

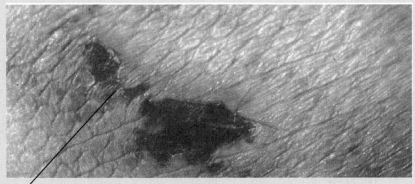

Cl: Hemorrhagic superficial necrosis.

Superficial
necrosis

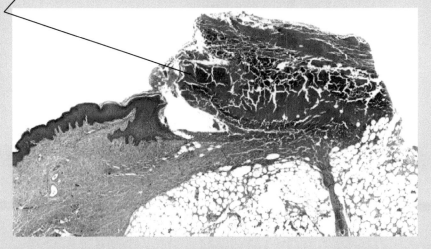

Vascular
changes

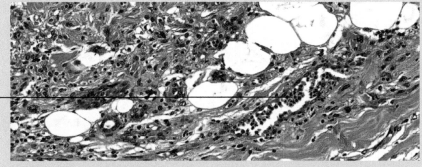

Hi: Fibrin and platelet thrombi. In advanced stages haemorrhage, necrosis en masse and ulceration. No significant vasculitis and inflammation.

DIFFERENTIAL DIAGNOSIS: Cryoglobulinemia type 1 (monoclonal type)

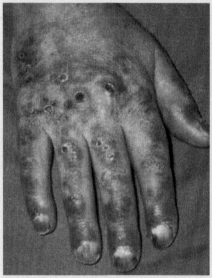
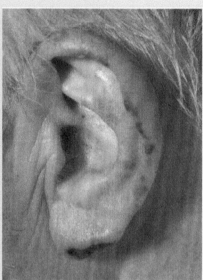

Acral livid infiltrates with superficial ulceration

Cl: Acral livid infiltrates with tendency to superficial ulceration.

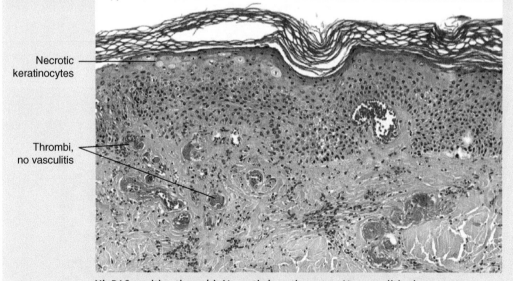

Necrotic keratinocytes

Thrombi, no vasculitis

Hi: PAS-positive thrombi. Necrotic keratinocytes. No vasculitic changes.

DIFFERENTIAL DIAGNOSIS: **Macroglobulinemia, (Waldenström, IgM)**

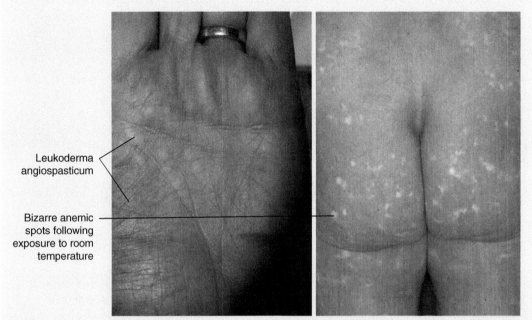

Leukoderma angiospasticum

Bizarre anemic spots following exposure to room temperature

Cl: Palms show white spots ("leukoderma angiospasticum"). Bizarre anemic spots in areas exposed to cold (room temperature).

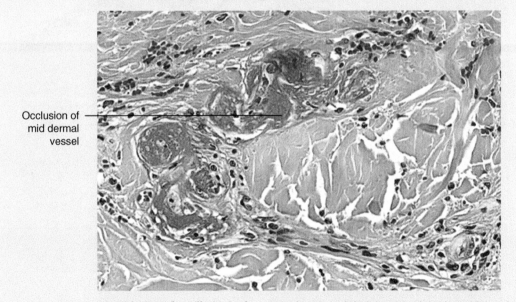

Occlusion of mid dermal vessel

Hi: Occlusion of capillaries in the upper dermis and draining vessels in the mid dermis.

DIFFERENTIAL DIAGNOSIS: Atrophie blanche (capillaritis alba)

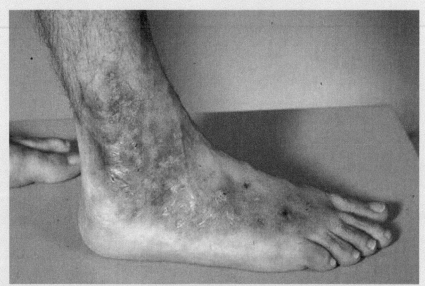

Atrophie blanche.
Capillaritis alba

CI: Atrophy, pigmentation due to hemosiderin deposits. Sclerosis, ulceration in advanced stages.

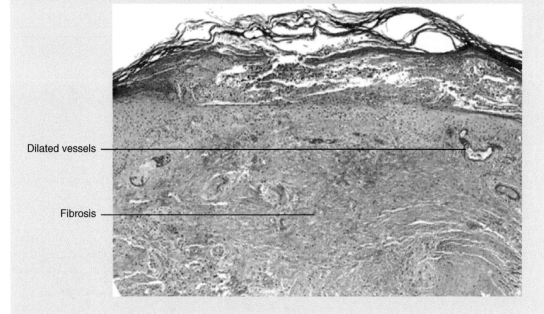

Dilated vessels

Fibrosis

Atrophie blanche (capillaritis alba)

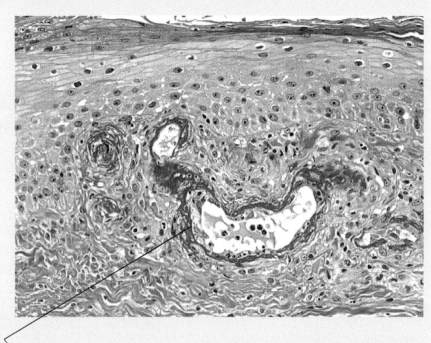

Dilated vessels with thickened vessel walls

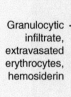

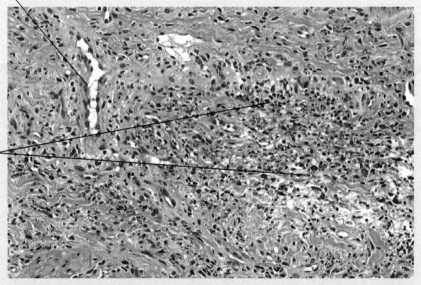

Granulocytic infiltrate, extravasated erythrocytes, hemosiderin

Hi: Fibrin thrombi in conjunction with fibrin rings in the vessel wall. No vasculitis. The combination of intravascular fibrin rings and thrombi is pathognomonic.

Atrophie blanche (capillaritis alba)

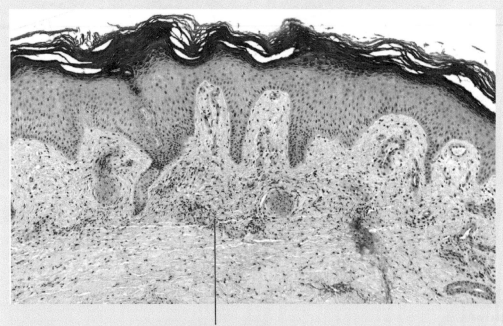

Thickening of vessel walls.
Fibrin rings (FITC, anti-fibrinogen)

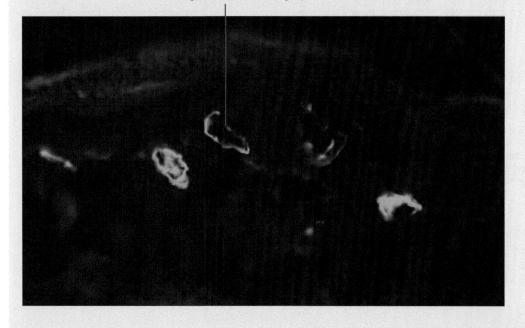

DIFFERENTIAL DIAGNOSIS: Malignant atrophic papulosis (Köhlmeier-Degos)

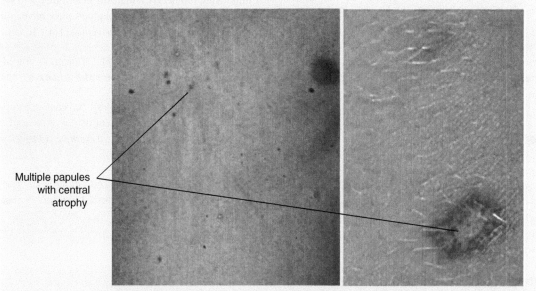

Multiple papules with central atrophy

Cl: Systemic disease involving skin, gut and central nervous system. Papules become centrally atrophic resulting in a white scar. No ulceration or crusts.

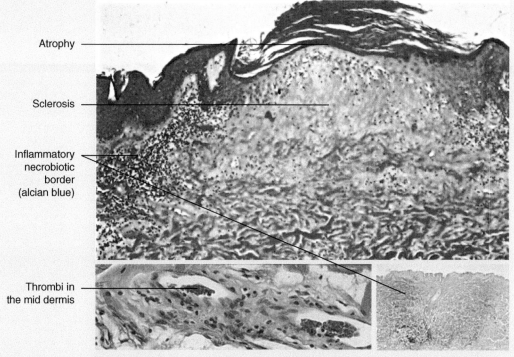

Atrophy

Sclerosis

Inflammatory necrobiotic border (alcian blue)

Thrombi in the mid dermis

Hi: Leukocytoklastic vasculitis with vascular occlusion in the deep dermis and wedge-shaped dermal necrosis.

Other Diagnosis

Thrombotic thrombocytopenic purpura (Werlhof disease): PAS-positive platelet-rich thrombi. No inflammation. No vasculitis. Erythrocyte extravasation of various degrees.

Antiphospholipid (Hughes) syndrome: thrombotic occlusion of arteries and veins due to hypercoagulability of the blood, caused by antiphospholipid antibodies.

Cutaneous cholesterol embolism: Occlusive vasculopathy with thrombi containing needle shaped cholesterol crystals (wedge-shaped open spaces).

References

Adcock, D. M., J. Brozna, *et al.* (1990). "Proposed classification and pathologic mechanisms of purpura fulminans and skin necrosis." *Semin Thromb Hemost* **16**(4): 333–40.

Burg, G., D. Vieluf, *et al.* (1989). "[Malignant atrophic papulosis (Kohlmeier-Degos disease)]." *Hautarzt* **40**(8): 480–5.

Gladson, C. L., P. Groncy, *et al.* (1987). "Coumarin necrosis, neonatal purpura fulminans, and protein C deficiency." *Arch Dermatol* **123**(12): 1701a–1706a.

Grilli, R., M. L. Soriano, *et al.* (1999). "Panniculitis mimicking lupus erythematosus profundus: a new histopathologic finding in malignant atrophic papulosis (Degos disease)." *Am J Dermatopathol* **21**(4): 365–8.

John, S., S. Manda, *et al.* (2011). "Cocaine-induced thrombotic vasculopathy." *Am J Med Sci* **342**(6): 524–6.

Papi, M., B. Didona, *et al.* (1998). "Livedo vasculopathy vs small vessel cutaneous vasculitis: Cytokine and platelet P-selectin studies." *Arch Dermatol* **134**(4): 447–52.

Thornsberry, L. A., K. I. LoSicco, *et al.* (2013). "The skin and hypercoagulable states." *J Am Acad Dermatol* **69**(3): 450–62.

PROTOTYPE: **Leukocytoklastic vasculitis**

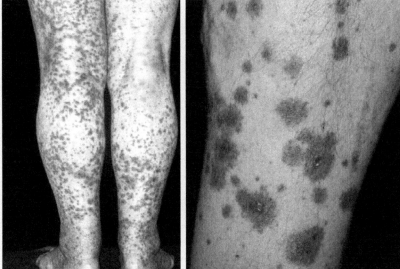

Purpura,
hemorrhagic
papules, necrosis

CI: Palpable purpura, hemorrhagic bullae, secondary necrosis; in some patients associated with internal involvement (kidney, GI tract, joints, nervous system) and corresponding symptoms.

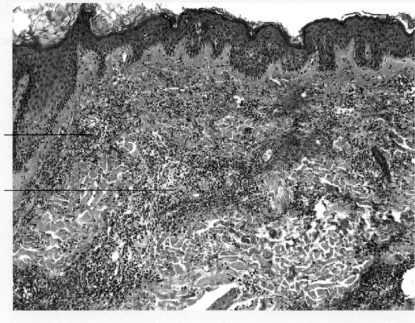

Destruction
of vessels

Mixed cellular
infiltrate

Leukocytoklastic vasculitis

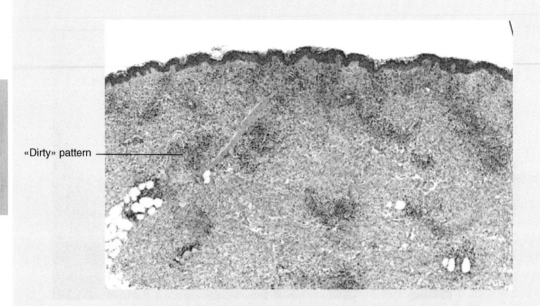

«Dirty» pattern

Small vessels with thickened walls (trichrome: fibrin and erythrocytes red)

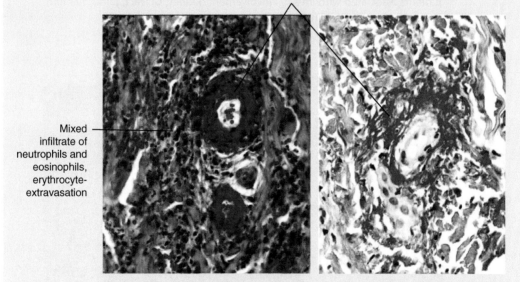

Mixed infiltrate of neutrophils and eosinophils, erythrocyte-extravasation

Hi: Damage of postcapillary venules in the dermis, patent lumina, destruction of vessel walls, intramural fibrin deposits, peri- and intravascular infiltrate with neutrophils and eosinophils, karyorrhexis with nuclear debris ("dirty" pattern), extravasation of erythrocytes, marked papillary edema, necrosis of overlying epidermis may occur.

Leukocytoklastic vasculitis

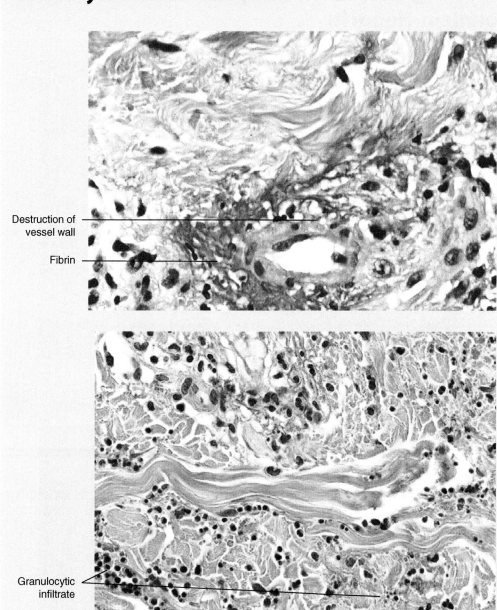

Destruction of vessel wall

Fibrin

Granulocytic infiltrate

VESSELS

VARIANT: IgA vasculitis (Purpura Schoenlein-Henoch)

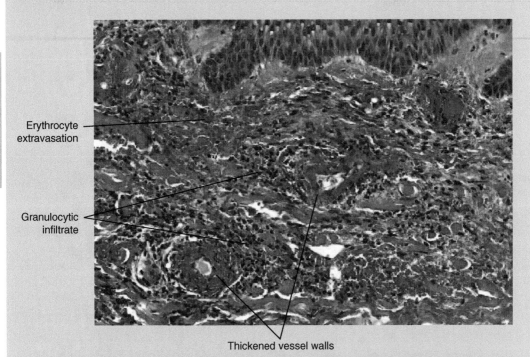

Erythrocyte extravasation

Granulocytic infiltrate

Thickened vessel walls

Cl: Purpuric hemorrhagic papules; systemic involvement (kidney, gut, joints).

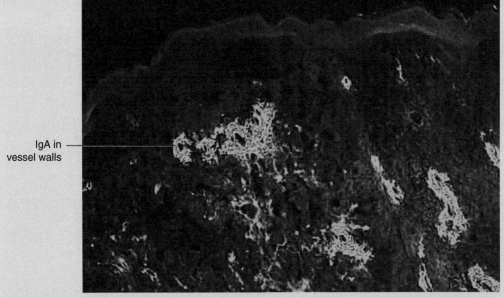

IgA in vessel walls

Hi: DIF: deposits of IgA in vessel walls. Involvement of visceral organs, especially GI tract and kidney.

VARIANT: **Bullous leukocytoklastic vasculitis**

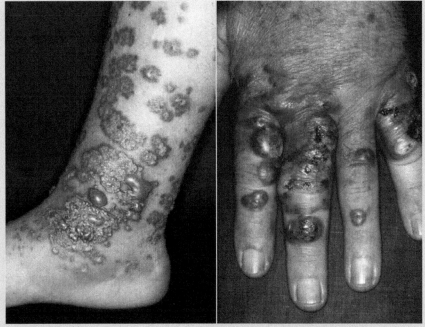

Bullae with
hemorrhage

Cl: Hemorrhagic bullae; hint for myelomonocytic and other leukemias.

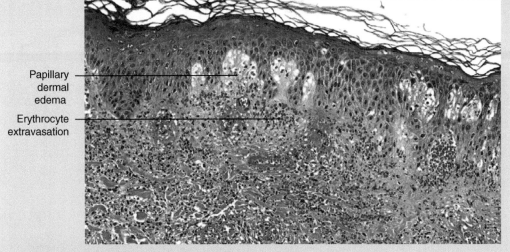

Papillary
dermal
edema

Erythrocyte
extravasation

Hi: Marked edema in the papillary dermis.

Pustular: with accumulation of neutrophils in the epidermis

Ulcerative: necrosis of the epidermis.

VESSELS

DIFFERENTIAL DIAGNOSIS: **Livedo racemosa**

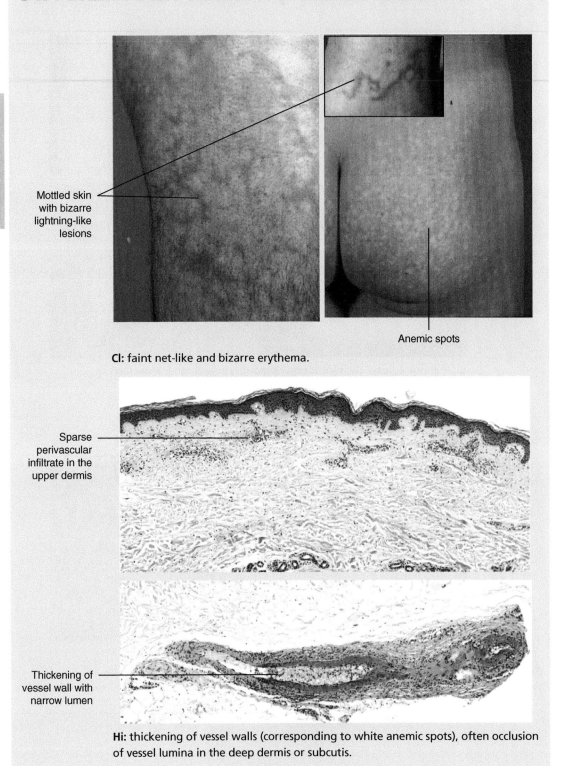

Mottled skin with bizarre lightning-like lesions

Anemic spots

CI: faint net-like and bizarre erythema.

Sparse perivascular infiltrate in the upper dermis

Thickening of vessel wall with narrow lumen

Hi: thickening of vessel walls (corresponding to white anemic spots), often occlusion of vessel lumina in the deep dermis or subcutis.

Other Diagnosis

Urticarial vasculitis (see Chapter 4, Edema, page 136*): Edema of the papillary and reticular dermis, perivascular and interstitial infiltrate of eosinophils and neutrophils, mild leukocytoklastic vasculitis, subtle or absent extravasation of erythrocytes.*

Septic vasculitis (Neisseria meningitidis, Staphylococci) (see Intravascular coagulation, page 224*): Necrosis of vessel walls, completely occluded, thrombosed lumina, nuclear dust, bacteria, occlusion of blood vessels by fibrin thrombi.*

Cryoglobulinemia (see Intravascular coagulation, page 226*): Fibrin thrombi only in type 1, leukocytoklastic vasculitis in type 2.*

Acute systemic lupus erythematosus (see Chapter 3, Lichenoid, page 117*): Interface dermatitis, lymphocytic nuclear dust.*

Papulosis maligna (Köhlmeier-Degos) (see Intravascular coagulation, page 231*): Leukocytoklastic vasculitis with vascular occlusion and wedge-shaped dermal necrosis.*

References

Carlson, J. A. (2010). "The histological assessment of cutaneous vasculitis." *Histopathology* **56**(1): 3–23.

Crowson, A. N., M. C. Mihm, Jr., *et al.* (2003). "Pyoderma gangrenosum: a review." *J Cutan Pathol* **30**(2): 97–107.

Crowson, A. N., M. C. Mihm, Jr., *et al.* (2003). "Cutaneous vasculitis: a review." *J Cutan Pathol* **30**(3): 161–73.

Hodge, S. J., J. P. Callen, *et al.* (1987). "Cutaneous leukocytoclastic vasculitis: correlation of histopathological changes with clinical severity and course." *J Cutan Pathol* **14**(5): 279–84.

Hurwitz, R. M. and J. H. Haseman (1993). "The evolution of pyoderma gangrenosum. A clinicopathologic correlation." *Am J Dermatopathol* **15**(1): 28–33.

Narula, N., S. Gupta, *et al.* (2005). "The primary vasculitides: a clinicopathologic correlation." *Am J Clin Pathol* **124 Suppl**: S84–95.

Russell, J. P. and L. E. Gibson (2006). "Primary cutaneous small vessel vasculitis: approach to diagnosis and treatment." *Int J Dermatol* **45**(1): 3–13.

Ryan, T. J. (1985). "Cutaneous vasculitis." *J Cutan Pathol* **12**(3–4): 381–7.

Su, W. P., A. L. Schroeter, *et al.* (1986). "Histopathologic and immunopathologic study of pyoderma gangrenosum." *J Cutan Pathol* **13**(5): 323–30.

PROTOTYPE: Cutaneous polyarteritis nodosa

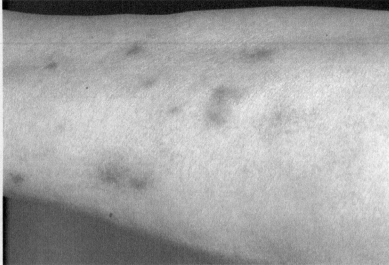

Multiple nodules

Cl: There is a broad spectrum of systemic manifestations due to infarction of specific organs, especially kidneys. In the skin painful erythematous nodules or ulcers which may be associated with subtle pattern of livedo reticularis.

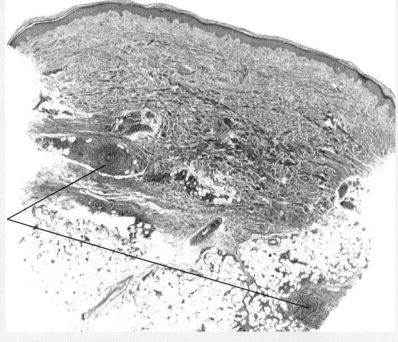

Thickened and almost occluded arterial vessels

Cutaneous polyarteritis nodosa

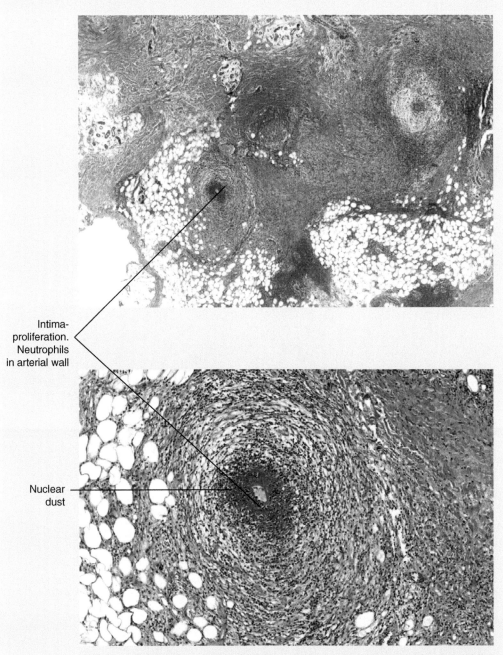

Intima-
proliferation.
Neutrophils
in arterial wall

Nuclear
dust

Hi: Leukocytoklastic vasculitis of small to medium-sized arteries with neutrophils, eosinophils, nuclear dust, fibrin in the vessel wall, intima proliferation and thrombotic occlusion of the lumen, occasional necrosis with ulceration. Elastica stain highlights the lamina elastica interna of the arterial vessel.

VESSELS

Cutaneous polyarteritis nodosa

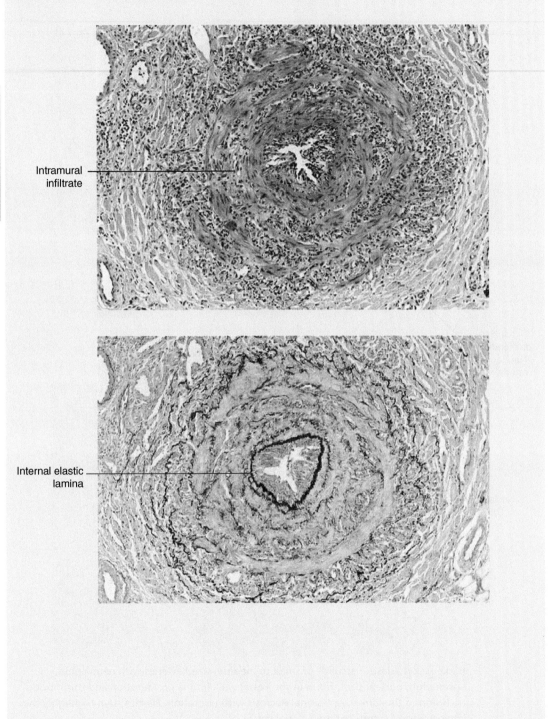

Intramural
infiltrate

Internal elastic
lamina

VARIANT

Microscopic polyarteritis: *necrotizing vasculitis, anti-neutrophil cytoplasmic autoantibodies (ANCA) frequently positive*

DIFFERENTIAL DIAGNOSIS

Superficial thrombophlebitis: Similar findings, but involvement of a vein

Wegener's granulomatosis: Leukocytoklastic vasculitis with granulomatous infiltrates. Pulmonary involvement in almost all patients.

Churg-Strauss syndrome (see page 165): Leukocytoklastic vasculitis with eosinophil rich infiltrates.

Nodular vasculitis: Lobular panniculitis with leukocytoklastic vasculitis of subcutaneous vessels

Comment

In individual cases it may be challenging to distinguish panarteritis nodosa from superficial thrombophlebitis on histological grounds alone.

References

Chen, K. R. (2010). "The misdiagnosis of superficial thrombophlebitis as cutaneous polyarteritis nodosa: features of the internal elastic lamina and the compact concentric muscular layer as diagnostic pitfalls." *Am J Dermatopathol* **32**(7): 688–93.

Hall, L. D., S. R. Dalton, *et al.* (2013). "Re-examination of features to distinguish polyarteritis nodosa from superficial thrombophlebitis." *Am J Dermatopathol* **35**(4): 463–71.

Ishibashi, M. and K. R. Chen (2008). "A morphological study of evolution of cutaneous polyarteritis nodosa." *Am J Dermatopathol* **30**(4): 319–26.

Marzano, A. V., P. Vezzoli, *et al.* (2013). "Skin involvement in cutaneous and systemic vasculitis." *Autoimmun Rev* **12**(4): 467–76.

VESSELS

PROTOTYPE: **Thrombophlebitis**

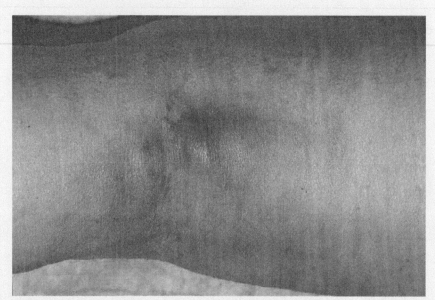

Erythematous
swelling

Cl: Distinct painful swelling with erythema and tenderness of the overlying skin, most frequently of the lower extremities. Multiple lesions may occur (so-called migratory thrombophlebitis).

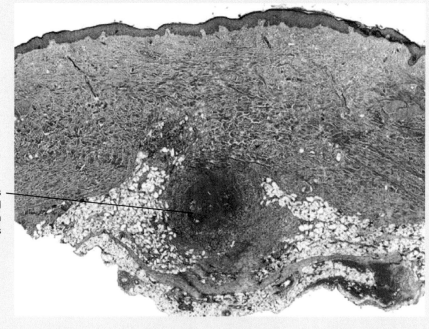

Subcutaneous
thick-walled
vein with
thrombus

Thrombophlebitis

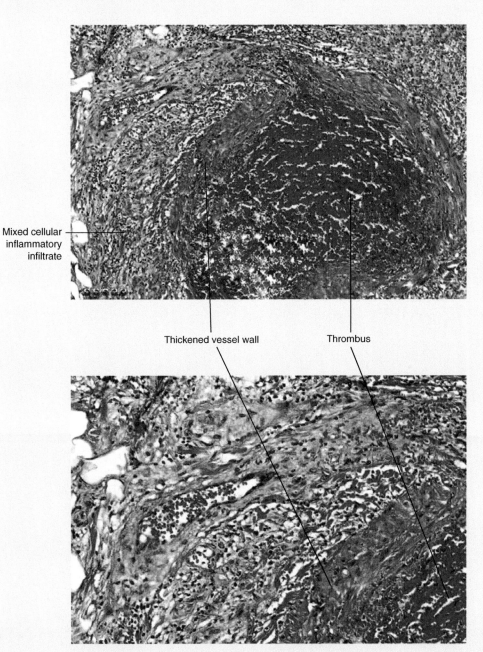

Mixed cellular inflammatory infiltrate

Thickened vessel wall · · · · · · Thrombus

Hi: Prominent vein in deep dermis or superficial subcutis with a thick muscular media and occluded lumen. Thrombus formation is paramount for the diagnosis of thrombophlebitis. Intramural inflammation may be scant, fibrinoid intramural deposits are absent. Early stages show neutrophil-rich infiltrates, mostly confined to the perivascular layers. Late stages show mixed inflammatory infiltrates surrounding the vessel but not spilling over into adjacent dermal or subcutaneous layers. Marked elastic fibers within thickened vessel wall.

VARIANT

Mondor disease: *distinct clinical features. Cord-like induration on the outer chest wall due to thrombophlebitis of the subcutaneous veins, always in linear arrangement.*

DIFFERENTIAL DIAGNOSIS

Polyarteritis nodosa (see Medium-sized vessels, page 240*): Marked intramural inflammation in conjunction with necrosis. Vasculitis mostly confined to arterioles (polyarteriolitis) of the deep dermis and superficial subcutis, but not to medium-sized or thicker arteries; the intramural inflammatory infiltrate widens the medial muscular arteriolar layer, thereby creating the false impression of a medium-sized thick-walled artery. A histopathological hallmark of polyarteritis nodosa is the patent vessel lumen in conjunction with dense intramural inflammation. There are typical intramural fibrinoid deposits forming a thick homogeneous ring between the intima and the lamina elastic interna.*

Nodular vasculitis: In many cases, deep thrombophlebitis is mistaken for nodular vasculitis, particularly in lesions involving the lower extremities. Classic nodular vasculitis involves medium-sized arteries of the subcutis with a dense infiltrate spilling over into adjacent tissues, e.g. the septa of the subcutaneous fat and the lobular fat.

Comment

As a *diagnostic clue*, nodular vasculitis presents with a thickened vessel wall devoid of elastic fibers between smooth muscle layers, while thrombophlebitis is characterized by multiple elastic fibers within the muscular vessel wall. Lamina elastica interna may be similar in both thick caliber veins and arteries of the lower limb.

VESSELS

Comments

The most challenging task in pathology of medium-sized vessel vasculitis is to differentiate between superficial thrombophlebitis of the lower extremities and cutaneous polyarteritis nodosa. It is quite remarkable that veins of the lower extremities are thick-walled, sometimes suggesting the pattern of mid-sized arteries. However, the muscular medial layer of thick-walled veins of lower extremities is multi-layered and includes multiple delicate strands of elastic fibers, while in mid-sized arteries there is a thick homogeneous and contiguous muscular layer without interspersed elastic fibers. Thrombophlebitis is always associated with thrombosed lumina, while in polyarteritis nodosa lumina are patent. The latter shows marked intramural inflammation with widening of the vessel wall and necrosis, while thrombophlebitis mostly is accompanied by a perivascular infiltrate confined to the immediate vicinity of the vessel. Fibrinoid deposits do not occur in vessel walls of thrombophlebitic lesions, but are quite characteristic of polyarteritis nodosa.

References

Alcaraz, I., J. M. Revelles, *et al.* (2010). "Superficial thrombophlebitis: A new clinical manifestation of the immune reconstitution inflammatory syndrome in a patient with HIV infection." *Am J Dermatopathol* **32**(8): 846–9.

Chen, K. R. (2010). "The misdiagnosis of superficial thrombophlebitis as cutaneous polyarteritis nodosa: features of the internal elastic lamina and the compact concentric muscular layer as diagnostic pitfalls." *Am J Dermatopathol* **32**(7): 688–93.

Hall, L. D., S. R. Dalton, *et al.* (2013). "Re-examination of features to distinguish polyarteritis nodosa from superficial thrombophlebitis." *Am J Dermatopathol* **35**(4): 463–71.

Yus, E. S., R. S. Simon, *et al.* (2012). "Vein, artery, or arteriole? A decisive question in hypodermal pathology." *Am J Dermatopathol* **34**(2): 229–32.

PROTOTYPE: **Erythema elevatum diutinum**

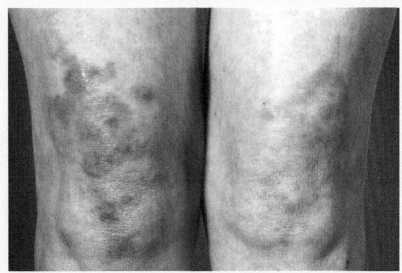

Pad-like
violaceous
plaques

Cl: Persistent, pad-like violaceous papules or plaques, symmetrically on the extensor surface of extremities.

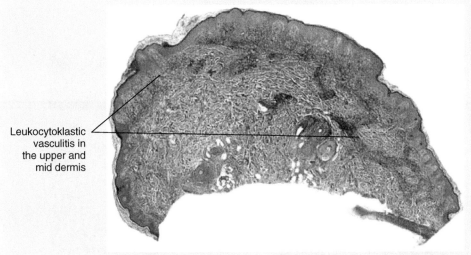

Leukocytoklastic
vasculitis in
the upper and
mid dermis

Hi: Leukocytoklastic vasculitis of small vessels in the upper and mid dermis with admixture of eosinophils and plasma cells and variable degrees of concentric fibrosis.

Early stage: Mixed cellular infiltrate. Lymphocytes, neutrophils, eosinophils, nuclear dust and leukocytoklastic vasculitis in the center of the infiltrates

Late stage: Concentric fibrosis, histiocytes and plasma cells.

VESSELS

VARIANT: **Granuloma faciale**

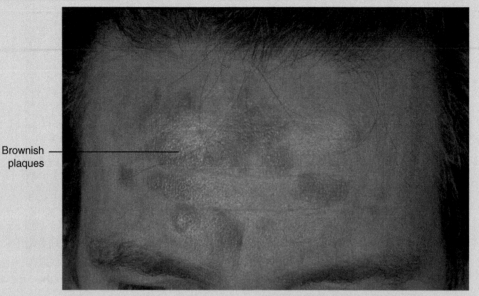

Brownish plaques

CI: Violaceous brown-red infiltrated plaque, preferentially in men's faces.

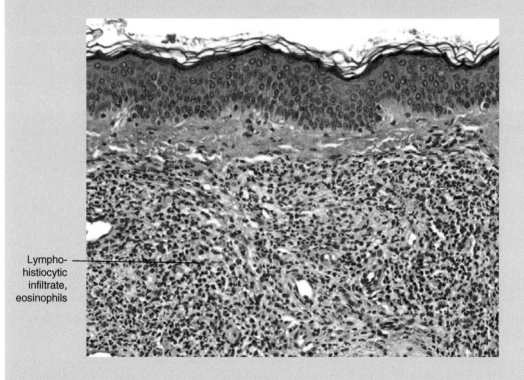

Lympho-histiocytic infiltrate, eosinophils

Granuloma faciale

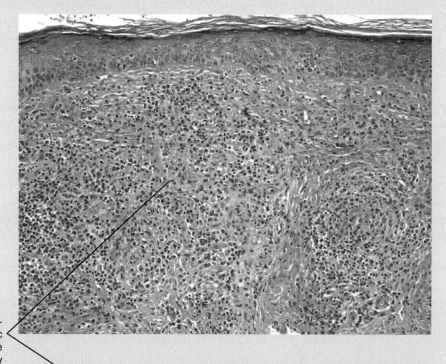

Lympho-
histiocytic
infiltrate
with many
eosinophils

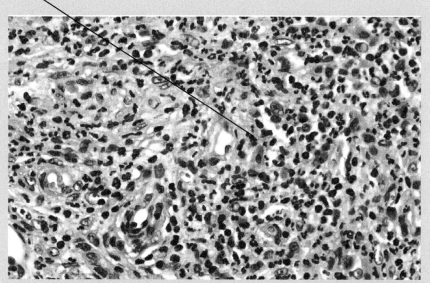

Hi: Overlapping with erythema elevatum et diutinum. There is a lymphohistiocytic ("granulomatous") infiltrate with leukocytoklasic vasculitis. Many eosinophils are present. Nuclear dust. Admixture of plasma cells.

DIFFERENTIAL DIAGNOSIS

Interstitial granulomatous dermatitis (see page 177*): Clinically shows patchy confluent erythema associated with arthritis. Histologically there is diffuse neutrophilic infiltrate, which tends to accumulate in dermal papillae; plasma cells.*

Sweet's syndrome (see Chapter 4, Non-granulomatous infiltrates, neutrophil- or eosinophil-rich, page 157*): Diffuse dermal neutrophilic infiltrate, no admixture of plasma cells, no prominent vasculitic features.*

Eosinophilic cellulitis (Wells syndrome) (see Chapter 4, Non-granulomatous infiltrates, eosinophil-rich, page 159*): Diffuse dermal infiltrates of eosinophils, flame figures, no vasculitis.*

Behçet's disease (see Chapter 2, Pustular, page 76*): In early stage: necrotizing leukocytoklastic vasculitis (pustules); Late stage: granulomatous reaction*

Comment

Erythema elevatum diutinum and granuloma faciale differ in regard to their clinical presentation, but show overlapping histological features. Therefore some experts consider the two conditions to represent one nosologic entity.

References

Caputo, R. and E. Alessi (1984). "Unique aspects of a lesion of erythema elevatum diutinum." *Am J Dermatopathol* **6**(5): 465–9.

Crowson, A. N., M. C. Mihm, Jr., *et al.* (2003). "Cutaneous vasculitis: a review." *J Cutan Pathol* **30**(3): 161–73.

Gibson, L. E. and R. A. el-Azhary (2000). "Erythema elevatum diutinum." *Clin Dermatol* **18**(3): 295–9.

Gibson, L. E. and W. P. Su (1995). "Cutaneous vasculitis." *Rheum Dis Clin North Am* **21**(4): 1097–1113.

LeBoit, P. E., T. S. Yen, *et al.* (1986). "The evolution of lesions in erythema elevatum diutinum." *Am J Dermatopathol* **8**(5): 392–402.

Lowe, L., B. Kornfeld, *et al.* (1992). "Rheumatoid neutrophilic dermatitis." *J Cutan Pathol* **19**(1): 48–53.

Ramsey, M. L., B. Gibson, *et al.* (1984). "Erythema elevatum diutinum." *Cutis* **34**(1): 41–3.

Sangueza, O. P., B. Pilcher, *et al.* (1997). "Erythema elevatum diutinum: a clinicopathological study of eight cases." *Am J Dermatopathol* **19**(3): 214–22.

Smoller, B. R., N. S. McNutt, *et al.* (1990). "The natural history of vasculitis. What the histology tells us about pathogenesis." *Arch Dermatol* **126**(1): 84–9.

Sunderkotter, C. (2013). "[Skin manifestations of different forms of vasculitis]." *Z Rheumatol* **72**(5): 436–44.

Wahl, C. E., M. B. Bouldin, *et al.* (2005). "Erythema elevatum diutinum: clinical, histopathologic, and immunohistochemical characteristics of six patients." *Am J Dermatopathol* **27**(5): 397–400.

Ziemer, M., M. J. Koehler, *et al.* (2011). "Erythema elevatum diutinum - a chronic leukocytoclastic vasculitis microscopically indistinguishable from granuloma faciale?" *J Cutan Pathol* **38**(11): 876–83.

PROTOTYPE: **Temporal arteritis**

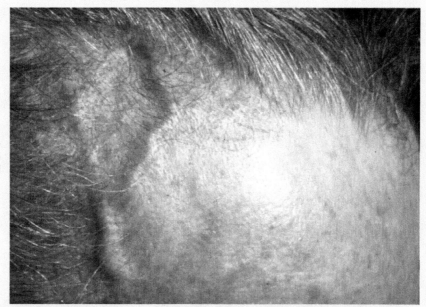

Palpable
arteria on
the forehead

Cl: Mostly in the temporal area erythema and ulceration overlying a palpable arteria. General symptoms include fever, pain and malaise. Sudden visual impairment may occur.

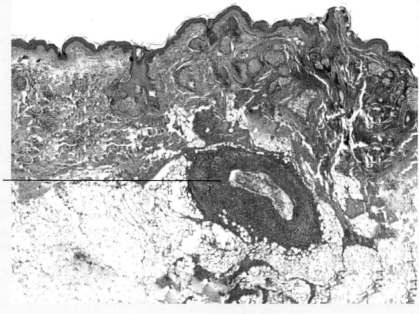

Temporal
artery

Temporal arteritis

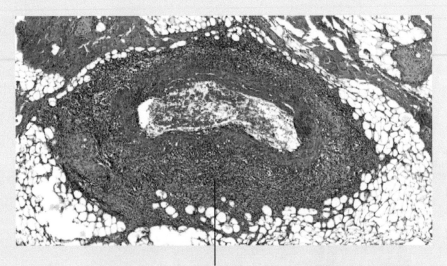

Mixed cellular infiltrate in the media of the vessel wall

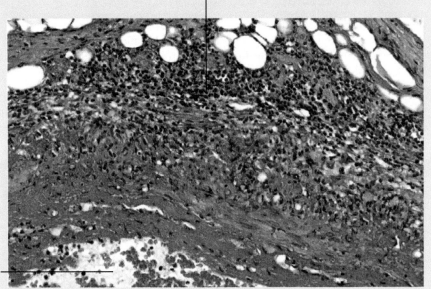

Vessel lumen

Hi: Granulomatous vasculitis involving medium to large arteries, with prominent skip areas. Vascular changes predominate in the inner media of the vessel wall with a mixed infiltrate containing multinucleated histiocytes. Destruction of the internal elastic lamina. No extravascular granuloma formation. Inflammatory changes may be restricted to the sub-intimal compartment of the vessel wall.

Temporal arteritis

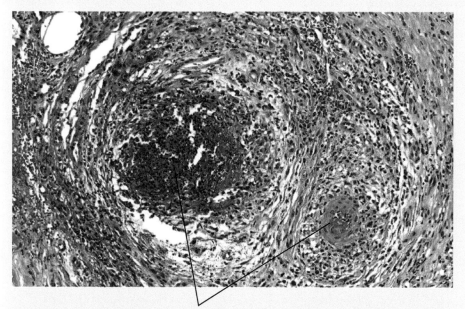

Destruction and occlusion of artery by mixed cellular inflammatory infiltrate

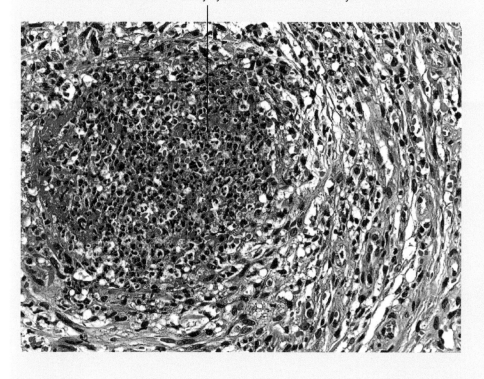

VARIANTS

Subintimal inflammatory changes, sparing the media, without marked multinucleate cells. Focal fragmentation of the internal elastic lamina.

DIFFERENTIAL DIAGNOSIS

Polyarteritis nodosa (see Medium-sized vessel, page 240*): leukocytoklastic vasculitis of small to medium-sized arteries, fibrin deposits, leukocytoklasia, no giant cells within vessel walls.*

Churg-Strauss syndrome (see page 165): *Eosinophilic extravascular palisading granulomas in conjunction with eosinophilic vasculitis. Extravascular palisading granulomas may be a prominent feature.*

Wegener's granulomatosis: Granulomatous vasculitis with extravascular palisading granulomas. Neutrophilic granulocytes may predominate.

Thrombangitis obliterans (Buerger's disease): Cellular mixed inflammatory infiltrate within vessel wall. No granulomatous changes. Scant neutrophils.

Lymphocytic thrombophilic (macular) arteritis: Medium-sized vessel vasculitis with fibrinoid thrombi or rims within the vessel and vessel wall, lymphocytes and histiocytes.

References

Carlson, J. A. (2010). "The histological assessment of cutaneous vasculitis." *Histopathology* **56**(1): 3–23.

Carlson, J. A. and K. R. Chen (2007). "Cutaneous vasculitis update: neutrophilic muscular vessel and eosinophilic, granulomatous, and lymphocytic vasculitis syndromes." *Am J Dermatopathol* **29**(1): 32–43.

Lee, J. S., S. Kossard, *et al.* (2008). "Lymphocytic thrombophilic arteritis: a newly described medium-sized vessel arteritis of the skin." *Arch Dermatol* **144**(9): 1175–82.

VESSELS

VESSELS

PROTOTYPE: Cutaneous calciphylaxis (calcifying uremic arteriolopathy)

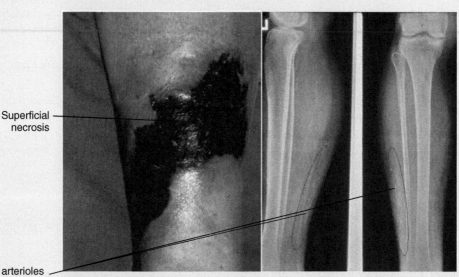

Superficial necrosis

Calcifying arterioles with faint contours

Cli: Superficial necrotic plaques and ulceration, usually on the lower leg in conjunction with chronic renal failure or/and hyperparathyroidism.

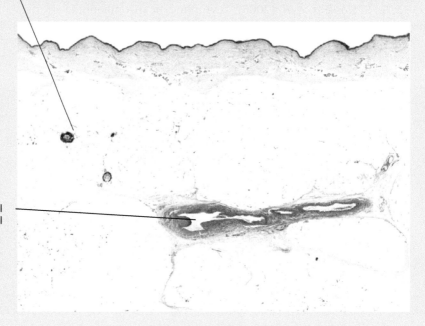

Dilated small vessel

Cutaneous calciphylaxis

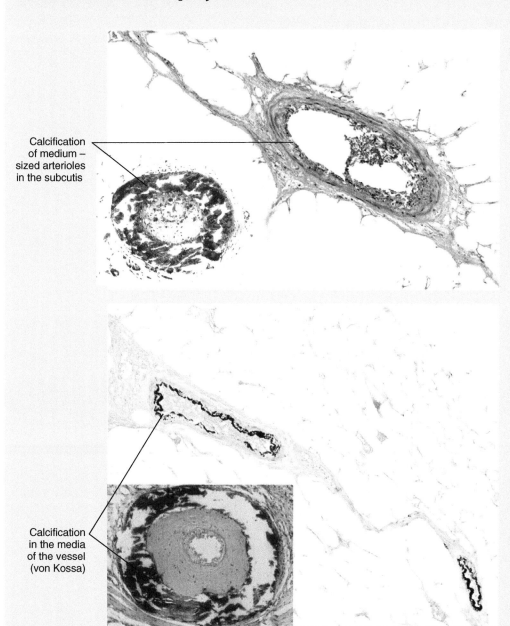

Calcification of medium – sized arterioles in the subcutis

Calcification in the media of the vessel (von Kossa)

Hi: cutaneous uremic calciphylaxis. The histopathological hallmarks of this condition are multiple tiny calcification foci within the subcutaneous fat, mostly in association with lobular capillaries and necrotic fat cells. Medial calcification of mid-sized arteries in conjunction with ulceration is common but cannot be used as a discriminating clue against Martorell's hypertensive arteriolosclerosis due to morphological overlap between the two entities.

VARIANTS

Early stage *may show only minimal calcification of vessels.*

Late stages *may be accompanied by massive inflammation and necrosis, simulating panniculitis or pyoderma gangraenosum.*

DIFFERENTIAL DIAGNOSIS

Arteriosclerosis: Incipient stages without visible clinical symptoms. Advanced stages with painful necrotic skin ulcers on the laterodorsal part of the leg, often with bilateral involvement. Ulcerations show morphological overlap with pyoderma gangraenosum. Systemic alterations include arterial hypertension and diabetes. Histology shows arteriolar changes in the deep dermis or subcutis with stenotic arteriolosclerosis and medial calcification, often in association with overlying ulceration. Arteriolar vessel walls are markedly thickened, with intramural medial calcification indistinguishable from calciphylaxis and other non-uremic variants of calciphylaxis. The ulceration may show undermined borders and a neutrophil-rich infiltrate, similar to histopathological changes in association with pyoderma gangrenosum. The condition is also known as Martorell's hypertensive ischemic leg ulcer.

Oxalosis: Birefringent crystalline deposits within lumina of small vessels. No significant vasculitic phenomena, no vessel wall calcification.

Non-uremic calciphylaxis: often indistinguishable from uremic calciphylaxis. Clinical investigations are paramount (calcium and phosphate levels, uremic parameters and others).

Cutaneous calcinosis: This multifactorial condition mostly affects the extravascular tissues. Significant vascular changes do not occur. Metaplastic calcification is typical of necrotic and tumorous foci.

Incidental calcification: Functionally insignificant vascular calcification indistinguishable from calcified arteriolosclerosis may be observed in the vicinity of excised epithelial or mesenchymal tumors from sun-exposed skin of the elderly, e.g. in BCC or SCC of the face.

VESSELS

Comment

The leading clinical picture with calcified arteriolosclerosis is Martorell's hypertensive ischemic leg ulcer, mostly affecting older patients with arterial hypertension and diabetes. Surprisingly, this condition is commonly confused with pyoderma gangraenosum, due to its massive ulceration. However, mural calcification of mid-sized arterial vessels is not an inherent part of pyoderma gangraenosum. Uremic and non-uremic calciphylaxis may be a significant pitfall in the diagnosis of subcutaneous arteriolosclerosis with vessel wall calcification. Remarkably, calcification of mid-mural myoid layers of arterioles are identical in both uremic/non-uremic calciphylaxis and in Martorell's calcified arteriolosclerosis. However, only the former conditions show conspicuous disseminated calcification in the subcutaneous fat with multiple calcified foci in association with capillaries between fat cells. Von Kossa stain may be necessary to appreciate these distinctive changes.

References

Edsall, L. C., J. C. English, 3rd, *et al.* (2004). "Calciphylaxis and metastatic calcification associated with nephrogenic fibrosing dermopathy." *J Cutan Pathol* **31**(3): 247–53.

Fernandez, K. H., V. Liu, *et al.* (2013). "Nonuremic calciphylaxis associated with histologic changes of pseudoxanthoma elasticum." *Am J Dermatopathol* **35**(1): 106–8.

Hafner, J., G. Keusch, *et al.* (1998). "Calciphylaxis: a syndrome of skin necrosis and acral gangrene in chronic renal failure." *Vasa* **27**(3): 137–43.

Hafner, J., G. Keusch, *et al.* (1995). "Uremic small-artery disease with medial calcification and intimal hyperplasia (so-called calciphylaxis): a complication of chronic renal failure and benefit from parathyroidectomy." *J Am Acad Dermatol* **33**(6): 954–62.

Hafner, J., S. Nobbe, *et al.* (2010). "Martorell hypertensive ischemic leg ulcer: a model of ischemic subcutaneous arteriolosclerosis." *Arch Dermatol* **146**(9): 961–8.

Lewis, K. G., B. W. Lester, *et al.* (2006). "Nephrogenic fibrosing dermopathy and calciphylaxis with pseudoxanthoma elasticum-like changes." *J Cutan Pathol* **33**(10): 695–700.

Mochel, M. C., R. Y. Arakaki, *et al.* (2013). "Cutaneous calciphylaxis: a retrospective histopathologic evaluation." *Am J Dermatopathol* **35**(5): 582–6.

Nikko, A. P., M. Dunningan, *et al.* (1996). "Calciphylaxis with histologic changes of pseudoxanthoma elasticum." *Am J Dermatopathol* **18**(4): 396–9.

Prinz Vavricka, B. M., C. Barry, *et al.* (2009). "Diffuse dermal angiomatosis associated with calciphylaxis." *Am J Dermatopathol* **31**(7): 653–7.

Solomon, A. R., S. L. Comite, *et al.* (1988). "Epidermal and follicular calciphylaxis." *J Cutan Pathol* **15**(5): 282–5.

Steele, K. T., B. J. Sullivan, *et al.* (2013). "Diffuse dermal angiomatosis associated with calciphylaxis in a patient with end-stage renal disease." *J Cutan Pathol* **40**(9): 829–32.

Zembowicz, A., P. Navarro, *et al.* (2011). "Subcutaneous thrombotic vasculopathy syndrome: an ominous condition reminiscent of calciphylaxis: calciphylaxis sine calcifications?" *Am J Dermatopathol* **33**(8): 796–802.

CHAPTER 6
Subcutis

Atlas of Dermatopathology: Practical Differential Diagnosis by Clinicopathologic Pattern, First Edition.
Edited by Günter Burg MD, Werner Kempf MD, and Heinz Kutzner MD. Co-Editors: Josef Feit MD, and Laszlo Karai MD.
© 2015 John Wiley & Sons, Ltd. Published 2015 by John Wiley & Sons, Ltd.

SUBCUTIS

PROTOTYPE: Erythema nodosum (early stage)

Bruise-like
swelling

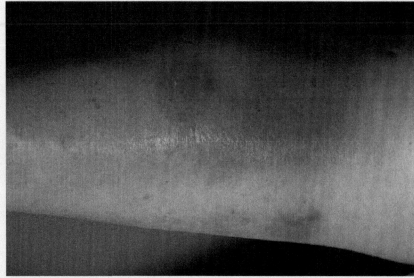

Cl: Bruise-like red, highly pressure sensitive swelling involving predominantly
the ankles, knees and anterior shins of middle-aged women. Ulceration does
not occur. Lesions heal within 4-8 weeks with complete regression without scars.

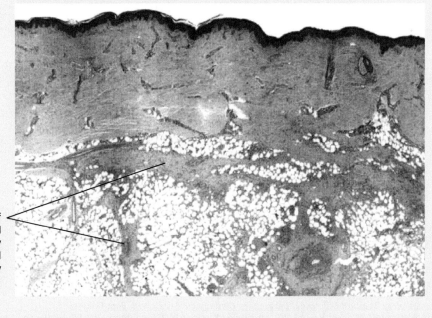

Thickening of
septae and
predominantly
septal
inflammatory
infiltrate

Erythema nodosum

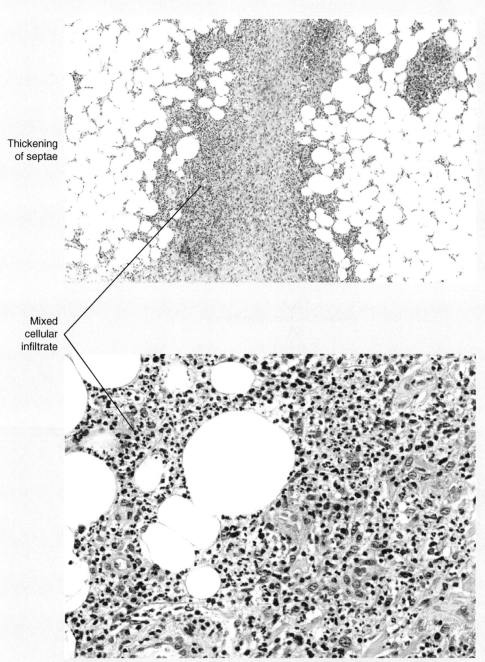

Thickening
of septae

Mixed
cellular
infiltrate

Hi: Thickening of subcutaneous septa, edema, neutrophils, eosinophils and lymphocytes (septal panniculitis), histiocytic granulomas in the periphery of fat lobules (Miescher's granulomas). No vasculitis.

Erythema nodosum

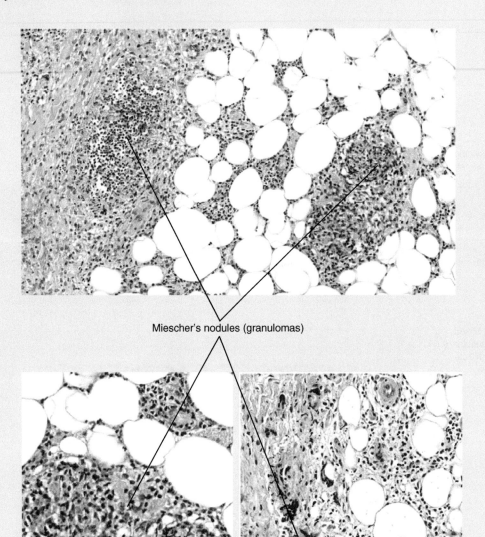

Miescher's nodules (granulomas)

DIFFERENTIAL DIAGNOSIS:

Septal panniculitis

Deep morphea: Thickened subcutaneous septa, subtle lymphocytic infiltrate with admixture of plasma cells.

Lobular panniculitis

Nodular vasculitis: Leukocytoklastic vasculitis involving venous and arterial vessels.

Erythema induratum Bazin (see Chapter 4, Granulomatous infiltrates, with necrosis)

Posttraumatic panniculitis: Foamy histiocytes surrounding pseudocystic spaces.

Factitial panniculitis

Infectious panniculitis: Septal and lobular mixed infiltrates with neutrophils, eosinophils and plasma cells. Abscess formation.

Comments

The clinical presentation in the various types of panniculitis uniformly is a more or less erythematous soft cushion-like swelling.

Erythema nodosum may occur in the context of sarcoidosis (Loefgren syndrome with hilar lymphadenopathy, polyarthritis and erythema nodosum).

References

Requena, L. and E. Sanchez Yus (2007). "Erythema nodosum." *Semin Cutan Med Surg* **26**(2): 114–25.

SUBCUTIS

SUBCUTIS

PROTOTYPE: Lupus panniculitis (Syn. Lupus profundus)

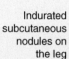

Indurated subcutaneous nodules on the leg

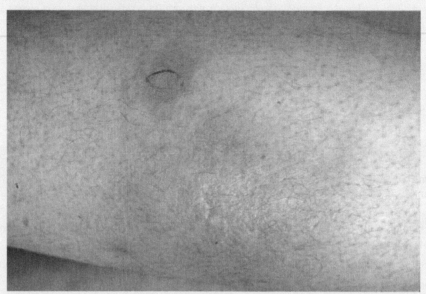

Cl: Multiple, subcutaneous indurated, painless nodules or plaques preferentially involving upper arms, shoulders, buttocks and breasts of women.

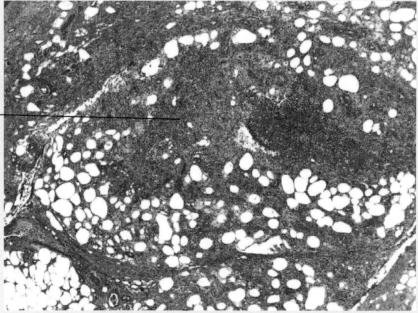

Lobular predominantly lymphocytic infiltrate

Hi: Lobular and paraseptal panniculitis with lymphocytic infiltrates and admixture of plasma cells and macrophages. Karyorrhexis. Mucin deposits in dermis and subcutis. No vasculitis. Rimming of adipocytes by lymphocytes, fat necrosis, plasma cells. No neutrophilic granulocytes.

DIFFERENTIAL DIAGNOSIS: Subcutaneous panniculitis-like T-cell lymphoma

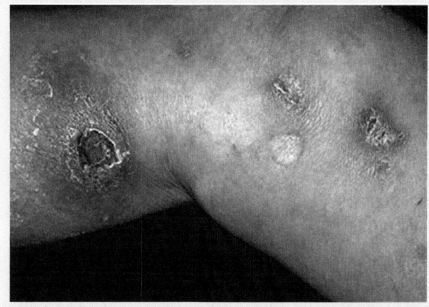

Ulcerated subcutaneous nodules

Cl: Multiple erythematous swelling and subcutaneous nodules without epidermal involvement except occasional occurrence of ulceration.

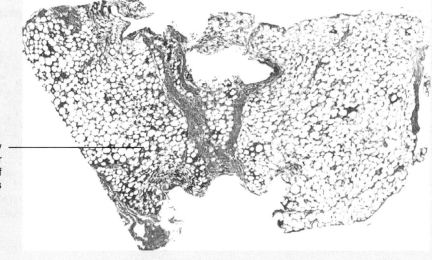

Predominantly lobular infiltrate of tumor cells

Subcutaneous panniculitis-like T-cell lymphoma

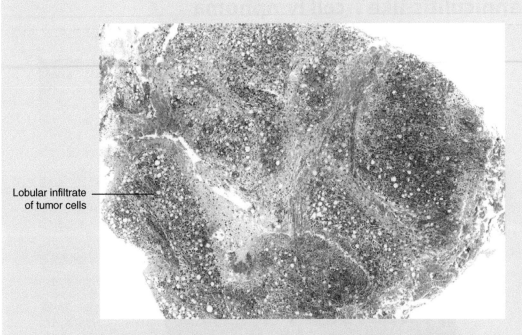

Lobular infiltrate
of tumor cells

Large anaplastic tumor cells

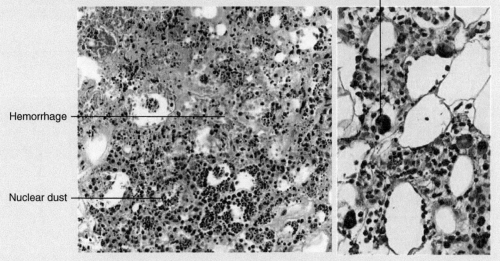

Hemorrhage

Nuclear dust

Hi: Lobular infiltrates of small to medium-sized lymphocytes with nuclear atypia which surround adipocytes (rimming). Lymphocytes express betaF1 and are CD8 positive. Large anaplastic tumor cells may occur in advanced stage.

DIFFERENTIAL DIAGNOSIS

Gamma/delta (γ/δ) T-cell lymphoma: range of lesions from subtle erythema, dermal/subcutaneous induration to (ulcerating) tumors. Histology: usually "three tiered" involvement of epidermis, dermis and panniculus. Tumor cells show similar features to **Subcutaneous panniculitis-like T-cell lymphoma** with more karyorrhexis, CD56 positive and gamma/delta phenotype (betaF1 is negative).

SUBCUTIS

DIFFERENTIAL DIAGNOSIS: **Paraffinoma**

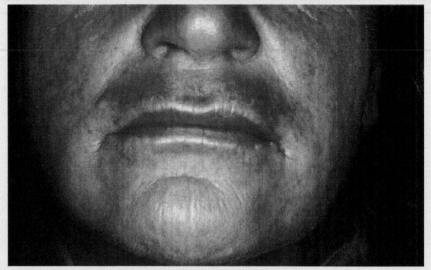

Swelling
of the upper lip

Cl: Swelling due to cutaneous and subcutaneous injections.

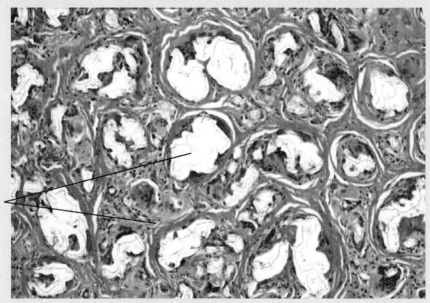

Bizarre clear
spaces and
fibrosis

Hi: Bizarre empty spaces within fibrotic tissue.

Other Diagnosis

Nodular vasculitis: Leukocytoklastic vasculitis, mostly lobular mixed infiltrate.

Erythema nodosum (*see* **page 268**)*: Septal infiltrates, mixed cellular in early stage, histiocyte-rich in late stage with granulomas (Miescher nodules).*

References

Massone, C., K. Kodama, *et al.* (2005). "Lupus erythematosus panniculitis (lupus profundus): clinical, histopathological, and molecular analysis of nine cases." *J Cutan Pathol* **32**(6): 396–404.

Park, H. S., J. W. Choi, *et al.* (2010). "Lupus erythematosus panniculitis: clinicopathological, immunophenotypic, and molecular studies." *Am J Dermatopathol* **32**(1): 24–30.

Requena, L. and E. Sanchez Yus (2001). "Panniculitis. Part II. Mostly lobular panniculitis." *J Am Acad Dermatol* **45**(3): 325–61; quiz 362–4.

SUBCUTIS

PROTOTYPE: Traumatic and factitious panniculitis

Indurated plaques, hemorrhage

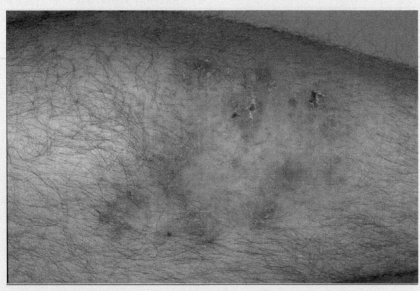

CI: Tender indurated plaques or nodules, after trauma or as a result of self-induced trauma.

Septal and lobular inflammatory infiltrate with hemorrhage

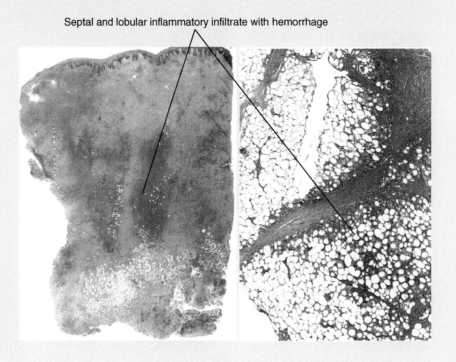

Traumatic and factitious panniculitis

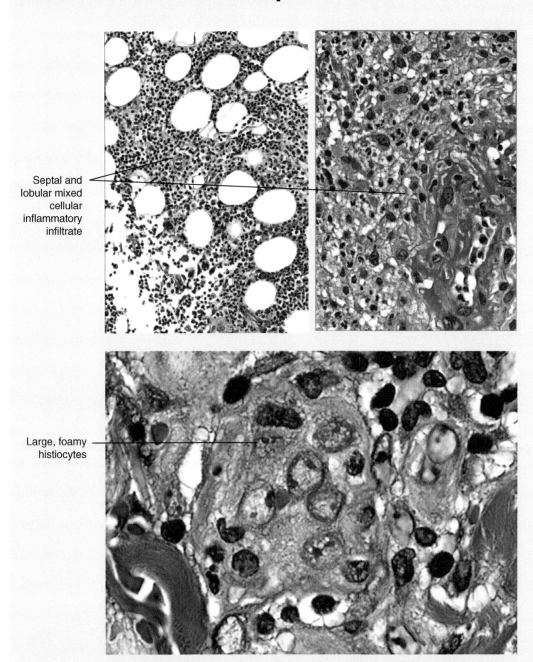

Septal and lobular mixed cellular inflammatory infiltrate

Large, foamy histiocytes

Hi: In the initial phase necrotic adipocytes, neutrophils and hemorrhage. In the later stage, foamy histiocytes within the lobules, pseudocyst formation due to necrosis of fat tissue, fibrosis. If the factitious panniculitis is associated with injection sometimes (polarizable or non-polarizable) foreign material can be identified.

SUBCUTIS

VARIANT

Subcutaneous fat necrosis of newborn: needle-like clefts

DIFFERENTIAL DIAGNOSIS: **Pancreatic panniculitis**

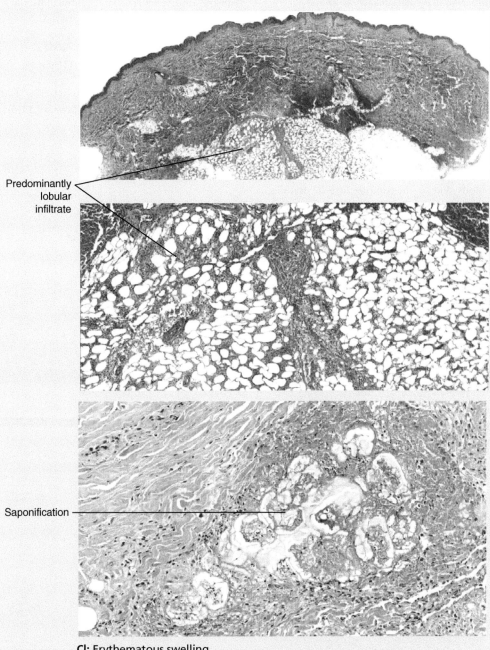

Predominantly lobular infiltrate

Saponification

CI: Erythematous swelling.

Hi: Lobular panniculitis with degeneration of the lipocytes and saponification (basophilic degeneration), infiltrate of neutrophils, lymphocytes and histiocytes surrounding necrotic adipocytes with thickened eosinophilic membranes (ghost cells).

Other Diagnosis

Infectious panniculitis: Mixed cellular infiltrate with abundant neutrophils in the septa and lobuli. Abscess formation may be present. Detection of microorganisms.

Alpha-1-antitrypsin deficiency: Ulcers draining oily material. Initially neutrophilic infiltrates in the reticular dermis, followed by septal and lobular infiltrates and necrosis. Later fibrosis and calcification.

Subcutaneous Sweet syndrome: diffuse subcutaneous infiltrates of neutrophils. No abscesses. Association with hematologic malignancies.

Comment

Many variations due to the various factitial injuries (trauma, injections).

References

Geraminejad, P., J. R. DeBloom, 2nd, *et al.* (2004). "Alpha-1-antitrypsin associated panniculitis: the MS variant." *J Am Acad Dermatol* **51**(4): 645–5.

Ter Poorten, M. C. and B. H. Thiers (2002). "Panniculitis." *Dermatol Clin* **20**(3): 421–33, vi.

Winkelmann, R. K. and S. M. Barker (1985). "Factitial traumatic panniculitis." *J Am Acad Dermatol* **13**(6): 988–94.

CHAPTER 7

Deposition and Storage

Atlas of Dermatopathology: Practical Differential Diagnosis by Clinicopathologic Pattern, First Edition.
Edited by Günter Burg MD, Werner Kempf MD, and Heinz Kutzner MD. Co-Editors: Josef Feit MD, and Laszlo Karai MD.
© 2015 John Wiley & Sons, Ltd. Published 2015 by John Wiley & Sons, Ltd.

PROTOTYPE: Tattoo

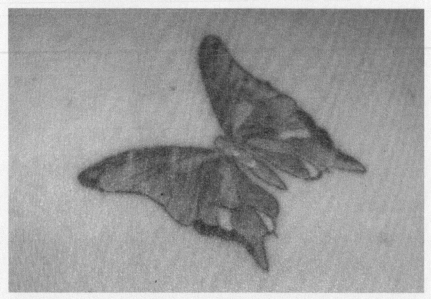

Cl: Permanent tattoos are made intentionally for cosmetic reasons or accidently (firecracker) by bringing a wide range of dyes and pigments into the dermal skin. They may lead to allergic reactions.

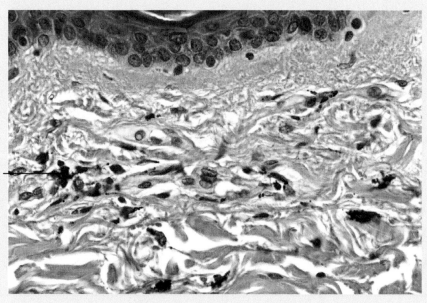

Intra-and extracellular pigment deposits

Tattoo

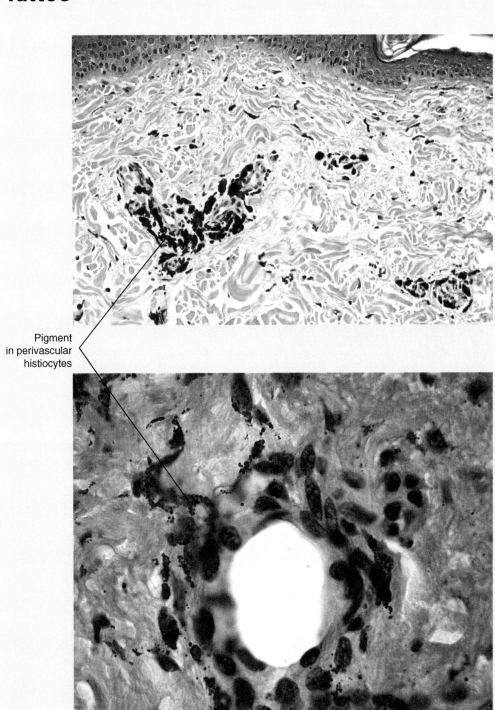

Pigment
in perivascular
histiocytes

Tattoo

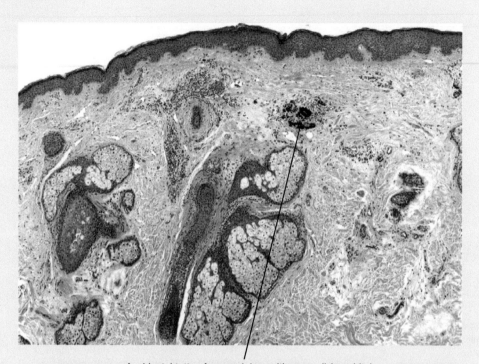

Accidental tattoo from an injury with a pencil (graphite)

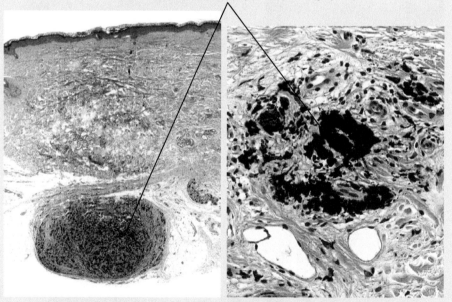

Hi: deposition of pigment extracellulary and in histiocytes of the upper and mid dermis, no or little inflammatory infiltrate.

VARIANTS

Eczematous reaction to tattoo dyes: Spongiosis.

Psoriasiform reaction.

Lichenoid and pseudolymphomatous reaction to tattoo: Interface dermatitis with band-like lymphocytic infiltrate. In addition, dense lymphocytic infiltrate in the deep dermis.

Granulomatous reaction: Sarcoidal granulomas, suppurative granulomas, necrobiotic areas.

Vasculitis: Small vessel leukocytoklastic vasculitis.

Fibrosing reaction: Histologically mimicking morphea.

DEPOSITION AND STORAGE

DIFFERENTIAL DIAGNOSIS: Erythema dyschromicum perstans

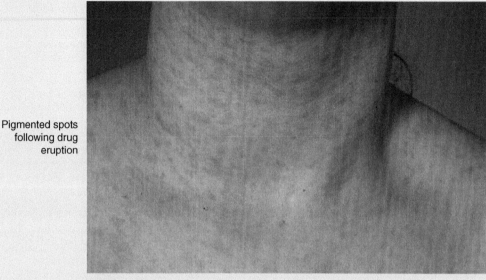

Pigmented spots following drug eruption

Cl: Brownish small patches.

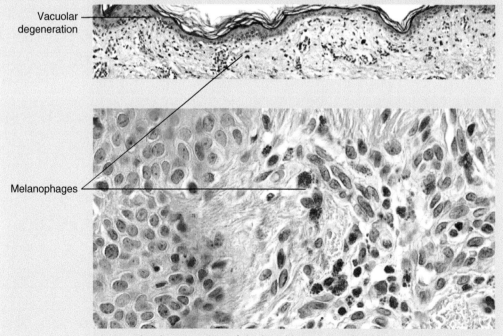

Vacuolar degeneration

Melanophages

Hi: Vacuolar degeneration of the basal layer, superficial lymphocytic infiltrate; scattered melanophages in the upper dermis.

DIFFERENTIAL DIAGNOSIS: **Blue nevus**

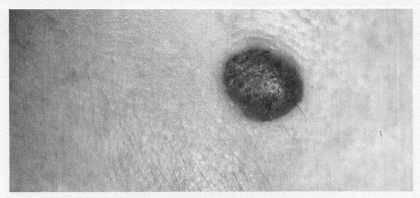

Cl: Black patch or nodule.

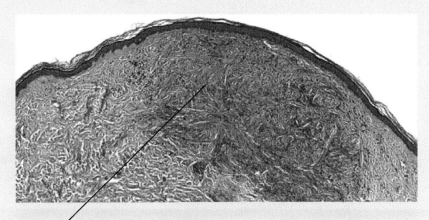

Aggregates of
melanocytes
and melanophages

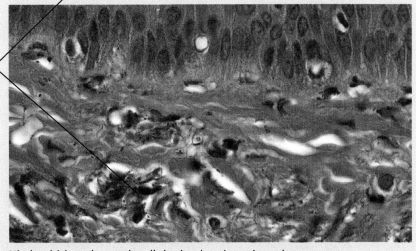

Hi: dendritic melanocytic cells in the dermis, melanophages.

DIFFERENTIAL DIAGNOSIS: Argyria

Normal hand

Greyish color in argyria

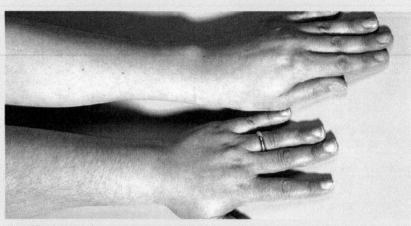

Cl: Diffuse bluish-brown discoloration.

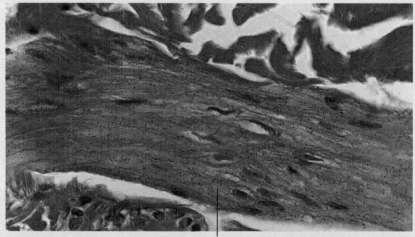

Faint «dirty» deposits of silver grains in elastic fibers around the fascia and the sweat glands

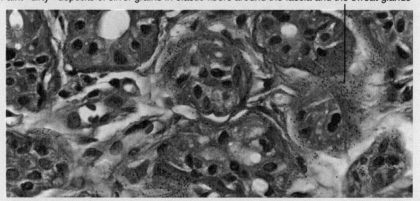

Hi: Deposits of silver at reticular fibers, especially around adnexal structures. No inflammatory infiltrate.

Other Diagnosis

Pigment incontinence following inflammation, due to friction or to melanosis in metastatic melanoma: granular melanin pigment mostly in macrophages (melanophages).

Amalgam deposits/Hydrargyrosis: Accidental amalgam deposits in the oral mucosa.

Ochronosis.

Comments

Epithelioid granulomas around tattoo may represent a local sarcoid reaction pattern to tattoo or represent cutaneous manifestation of systemic sarcoidosis.

Granulomatous reaction may represent complication by mycobacterial infection: Search for acid-fast bacilli by Ziehl-Neelsen stain or mycobacterial DNA by polymerase chain reaction.

References

Balfour, E., I. Olhoffer, *et al.* (2003). "Massive pseudoepitheliomatous hyperplasia: an unusual reaction to a tattoo." *Am J Dermatopathol* **25**(4): 338–40.

Mahalingam, M., E. Kim, *et al.* (2002). "Morphea-like tattoo reaction." *Am J Dermatopathol* **24**(5): 392–5.

Sweeney, S. A., L. D. Hicks, et al. (2013). "Perforating granulomatous dermatitis reaction to exogenous tattoo pigment: a case report and review of the literature." *Am J Dermatopathol* **35**(7): 754–6.

Thum, C. K. and A. Biswas (2014). "Inflammatory complications related to tattooing: A histopathological approach based on pattern analysis." *Am J Dermatopathol* **36**(3): e70–4.

Wenzel, S. M., I. Rittmann, *et al.* (2013). "Adverse reactions after tattooing: review of the literature and comparison to results of a survey." *Dermatology* **226**(2): 138–47.

DEPOSITION AND STORAGE

PROTOTYPE: **Xanthoma**

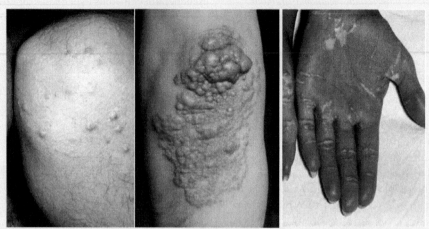

Eruptive xanthomas   Nodular xanthomas   Tendinous xanthomas

Cl: There are many different variants of xanthomas, which all show yellowish discoloration of the skin in the area of deposition of lipids. There may be flat lesions like in xanthelasma or nodular lesions of various sizes.

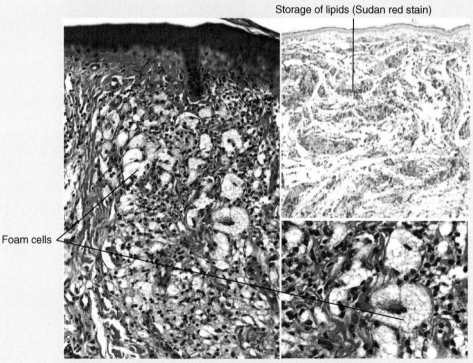

Hi: Clusters of foamy histiocytes; no or little inflammatory infiltrate; occasionally deposits of extracellular lipids.

VARIANTS: **Xanthelasma**

Yellow plaques

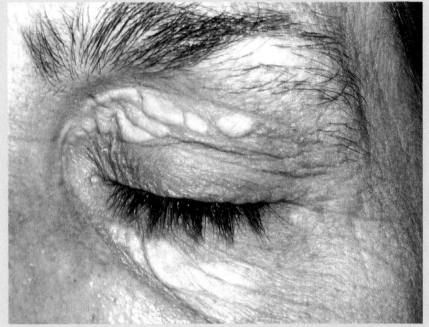

Cl: Yellow plaques periocularly.

Foamy cells

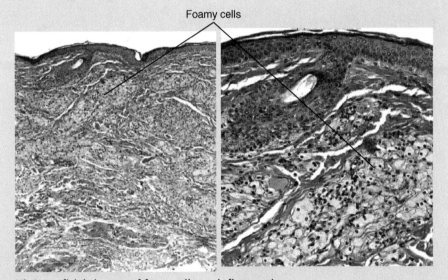

Hi: Superficial clusters of foam cells; no inflammation.

Variants:
   Tendinous xanthomas
   Eruptive xanthomas
   Nodular xanthomas

DIFFERENTIAL DIAGNOSIS: Verruciform xanthoma

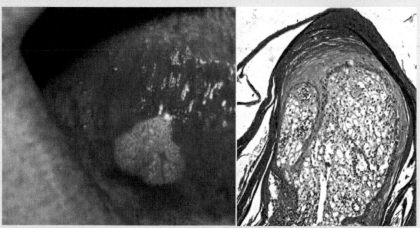

Nodule on
the tongue

Verruciform lesion (nose)

Cl: Solitary papular lesion, usually on the tongue, occasionally in the nostril.

Foam cells

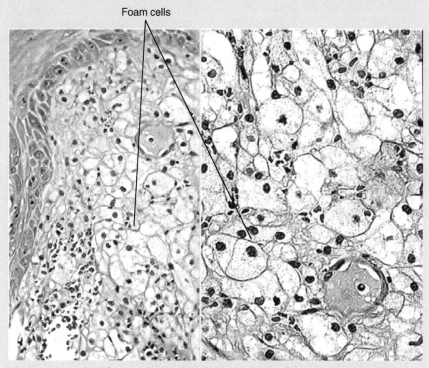

Hi: Densely packed foam cells are seen in the dermis of the verruciform lesion.

DIFFERENTIAL DIAGNOSIS: Necrobiotic xanthogranuloma

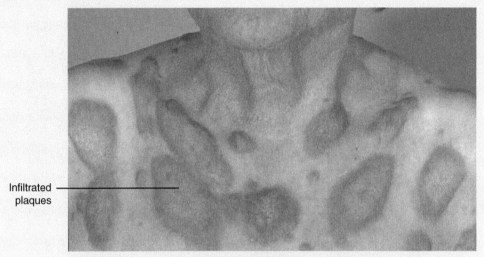

Infiltrated plaques

Cl: Mostly in association with IgG paraproteinemia. Yellowish indurated plaques.

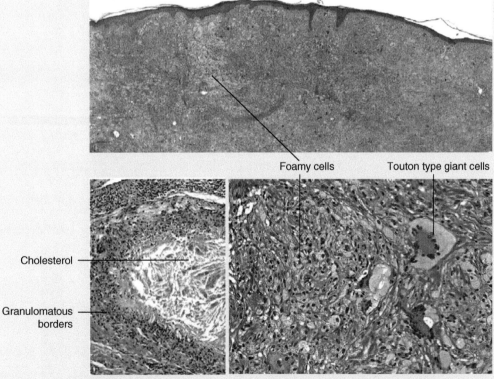

Foamy cells   Touton type giant cells

Cholesterol

Granulomatous borders

Hi: Large areas of collagen degeneration, sheets of foamy cells, cholesterol clefts and Touton type giant cells. Often prominent palisading.

Comment

May be nosologically identical with annular elastolytic giant cell granuloma (see DERMIS, Granulomatous, page 190).

DEPOSITION AND STORAGE

DIFFERENTIAL DIAGNOSIS: Axillary perifollicular xanthomatosis (Fox-Fordyce disease)

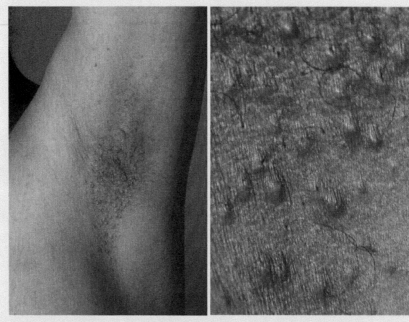

Follicular
papular
eruptions

CI: Follicular papular eruptions in the axillae.

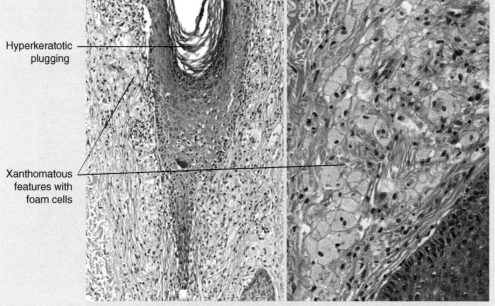

Hyperkeratotic
plugging

Xanthomatous
features with
foam cells

Hi: Hyperkeratotic plugging of the follicles, surrounded by inflammatory infiltrate and occasionally xanthomatous features.

Other Diagnosis

Juvenile xanthogranuloma (see Chapter 4,
Granulomatous infiltrates, Proliferative, page 199*):*
solitary or multiple papules. Histology shows a dense infiltrate
of macrophages with abundant slightly eosinophilic cytoplasm
in early lesions, whereas in mature lesions foamy cells and
Touton giant-cells are seen. Admixture of eosinophils.

References

Beham, A. and C. D. Fletcher (1991). "Plexiform
xanthoma: an unusual variant." *Histopathology* **19**(6):
565–7.

Bito, T., C. Kawakami, *et al.* (2010). "Generalized
eruptive xanthoma with prominent deposition of
naked chylomicrons: evidence for chylomicrons as the
origin of urate-like crystals." *J Cutan Pathol* **37**(11):
1161–3.

Breier, F., B. Zelger, *et al.* (2002). "Papular xanthoma:
a clinicopathological study of 10 cases." *J Cutan Pathol*
29(4): 200–6.

Cooper, P. H. (1986). "Eruptive xanthoma: a
microscopic simulant of granuloma annulare." *J Cutan
Pathol* **13**(3): 207–15.

Kossard, S. and P. Dwyer (2004). "Axillary
perifollicular xanthomatosis resembling Fox-Fordyce
disease." *Australas J Dermatol* **45**(2): 146–8.

Mete, O., E. Kurklu, *et al.* (2009). "Flat type
verruciform xanthoma of the tongue and its differential
diagnosis." *Dermatology Online Journal* **15**(9).

Molina-Ruiz, A. M., L. Cerroni, *et al.* (2014).
"Cutaneous Deposits." *Am J Dermatopathol* **36**(1): 1–48.

Williford, P. M., W. L. White, *et al.* (1993). "The
spectrum of normolipemic plane xanthoma." *Am J
Dermatopathol* **15**(6): 572–5.

DEPOSITION AND STORAGE

PROTOTYPE: Myxedema, diffuse, generalized

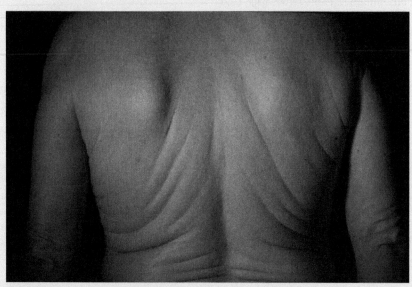

Waxy pale and thickened skin with typical skinfolds

Cl: Deposition of mucin in the dermis due to hypothyroidism leads to diffuse swelling and waxy pale and dry skin.

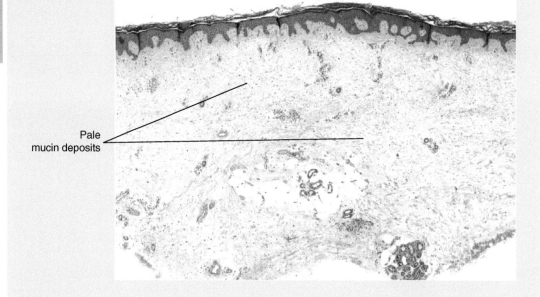

Pale mucin deposits

Myxedema

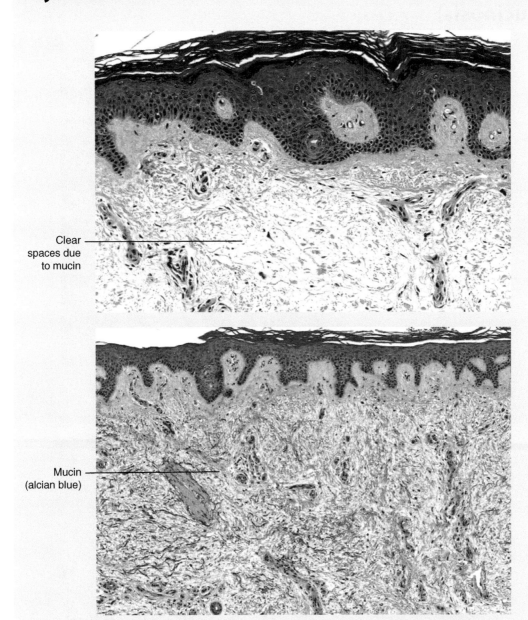

Clear spaces due to mucin

Mucin (alcian blue)

Hi: Hyperkeratosis, slight edema and abundant mucin, fibrosis in deep dermis and subcutis in late stages, simulating scleroderma.

VARIANTS: Lichen myxedematosus (papular mucinosis)

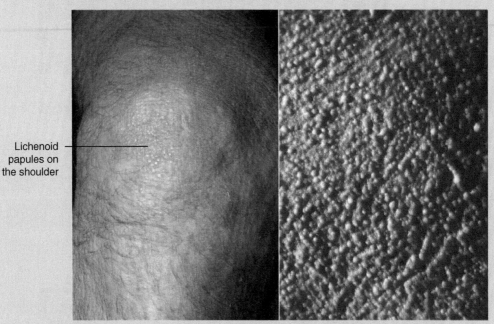

Lichenoid papules on the shoulder

Cl: Disseminated papules on hands or on extensor sites of the extremities.

Mucin deposits (HE, alcian blue)

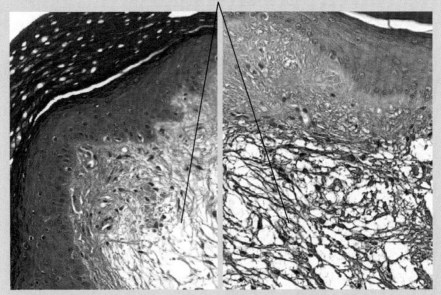

Hi: Thinning of the epidermis, flattening of rete ridges, atrophy of adnexal structures, diffuse deposits of mucin in the upper and mid dermis, dense packing of thickened collagen bundles (fibromucinosis), proliferation of fibroblasts, sparse lymphocytic infiltrate.

Praetibial myxedema: association with thyroid dysfunction

DIFFERENTIAL DIAGNOSIS: Scleromyxedema (Arndt-Gottron)

Lichenoid papules on the ball of the thumb

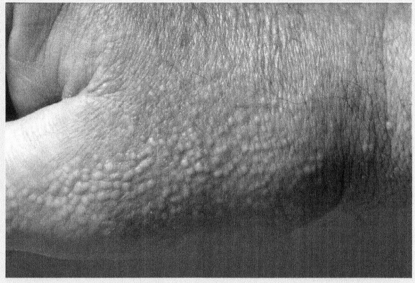

Cl: Lichenoid papules and diffuse elephant skin-like thickening with deep folds in tension lines. Association with underlying monoclonal gammopathy in some patients.

Mucin deposits (HE, alcian blue)

Increased number of fibroblasts

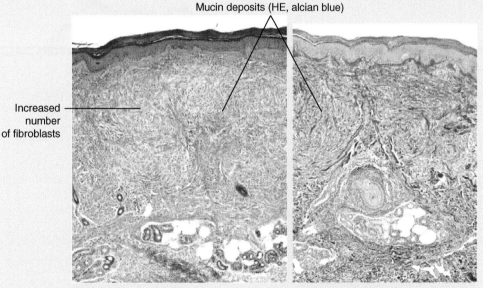

Hi: Deposits of mucin in the dermis, thickened collagen bundles, some plasma cells.

DEPOSITION AND STORAGE

DIFFERENTIAL DIAGNOSIS: Reticular erythematous mucinosis (REM)

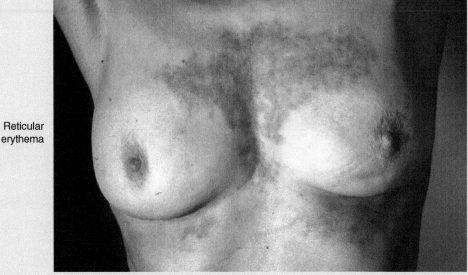

Reticular erythema

Cl: Fine reticular erythema, preferentially on the chest.

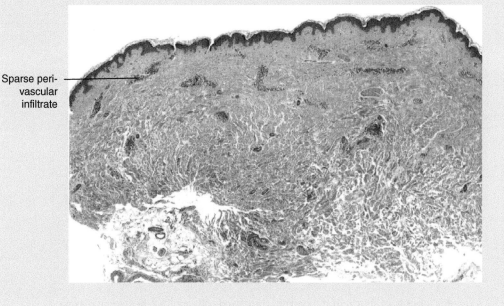

Sparse perivascular infiltrate

Reticular erythematous mucinosis (REM)

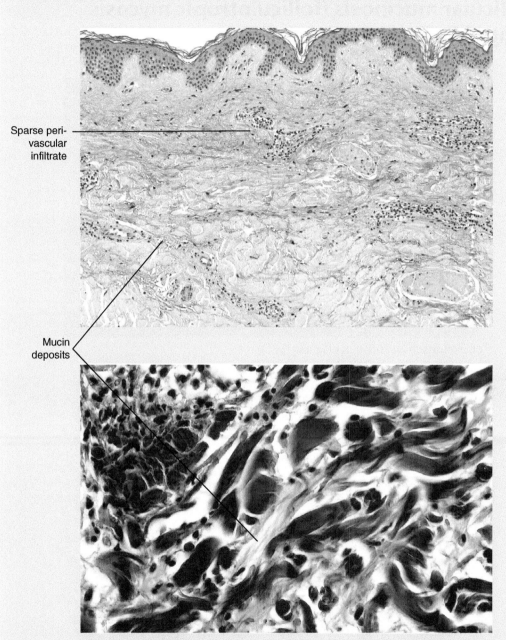

Sparse peri-vascular infiltrate

Mucin deposits

Hi: Normal epidermis, mucin in upper and mid dermis, sparse perivascular and periadnexal lymphocytic infiltrate.

DEPOSITION AND STORAGE

DIFFERENTIAL DIAGNOSIS: Lymphoma associated follicular mucinosis (folliculotropic mycosis fungoides)

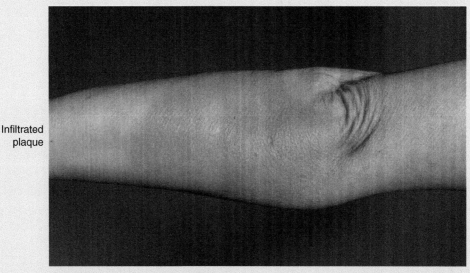

Infiltrated plaque

Cl: Infiltrated erythematous plaques.

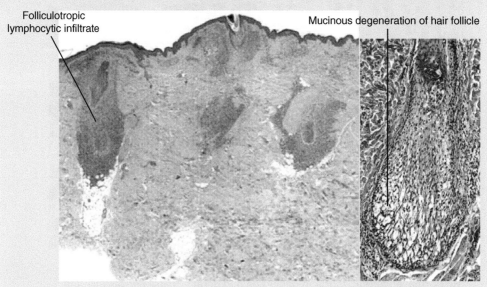

Folliculotropic lymphocytic infiltrate

Mucinous degeneration of hair follicle

Hi: Epidermo-and folliculo-tropic lymphocytic infiltrate. Mucinous degeneration of hair follicles.

DIFFERENTIAL DIAGNOSIS: **Mucoid pseudocyst of the digit or of the lip**

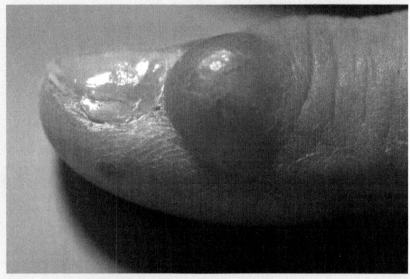

Cyst over distal interphalangeal joint

Cl: Translucent cystic lesion, frequently following injury.

Mucin deposits (HE, alcian blue)

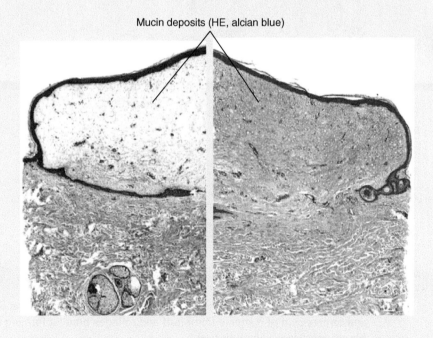

Mucoid pseudocyst

DEPOSITION AND STORAGE

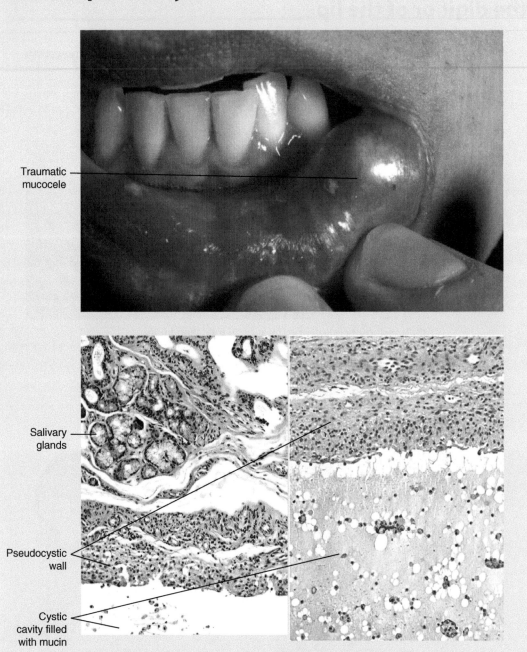

Traumatic mucocele

Salivary glands

Pseudocystic wall

Cystic cavity filled with mucin

Hi: Cavity filled with loose mucoid material; lack of epithelium; alignment and compression of marginal fibroblasts and collagen bundles forming a fibroconnective wall (pseudocyst).

DIFFERENTIAL DIAGNOSIS: **Cutaneous myxoma**

Cl: Circumscribed, soft nodular lesion.

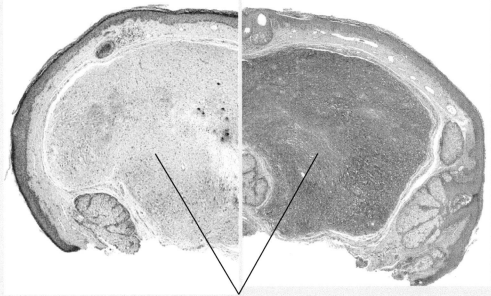

Well-defined, circumscribed, unencapsulated mucin deposits (HE, alcian blue)

Spindle-shaped and dendritic fibroblasts

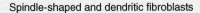

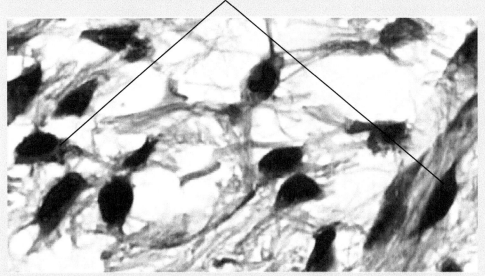

Hi: Unencapsulated, well-defined mucin deposition in the dermis and subcutis, increased number of myofibroblasts, smooth muscle-actin positive cells, factor XIII negative.

Other Diagnosis

Cutaneous focal mucinosis: Ill-defined mucin deposits in the dermis; smooth muscle-actin negative, factor XIIIa positive dendritic cells.

Scleroderma (see Chapter 4, Sclerosis, page 208*): thickened collagen bundles, no macrophages.*

Scleredema adultorum Buschke: Diffuse thickening of the skin due to deposits of mucopolysaccharides; "peau d'orange"-aspect; no increased number of fibroblasts; frequent association with diabetes.

Lupus erythematosus (see Chapter 4, DERMIS, Infiltrates, non-granulomatous, lymphocytic, page 142*): Sleeve-like perivascular and periadnexal lymphocytic infiltrate.*

Myxoid neurothekeoma: Well circumscribed lobulated proliferation of S100-positive spindled and epithelioid cells and myxoid stroma.

Comment

Histologically, ganglion and digital mucoid cyst cannot be distinguished.

References

Bolton, J. G. and E. K. Satter (2012). "An interstitial granulomatous pattern in localized lichen myxedematosus with associated monoclonal gammopathy." *J Cutan Pathol* **39**(3): 395–8.

Jackson, E. M. and J. C. English, 3rd (2002). "Diffuse cutaneous mucinoses." *Dermatol Clin* **20**(3): 493–501.

Kerns, M. J. and D. F. Mutasim (2010). "Focal cutaneous mucinosis in Graves disease: relation to pretibial myxedema." *Am J Dermatopathol* **32**(2): 196–7.

Li, K. and B. Barankin (2010). "Digital mucous cysts." *J Cutan Med Surg* **14**(5): 199–206.

Molina-Ruiz, A. M., L. Cerroni, *et al.* (2014). "Cutaneous deposits." *Am J Dermatopathol* **36**(1): 1–48.

Pomann, J. J. and E. J. Rudner (2003). "Scleromyxedema revisited." *Int J Dermatol* **42**(1): 31–5.

Rongioletti, F. and A. Rebora (2001). "Updated classification of papular mucinosis, lichen myxedematosus, and scleromyxedema." *J Am Acad Dermatol* **44**(2): 273–81.

Sonnex, T. S. (1986). "Digital myxoid cysts: a review." *Cutis* **37**(2): 89–94.

Takemura, N., N. Fujii, *et al.* (2005). "Cutaneous focal mucinosis: a case report." *J Dermatol* **32**(12): 1051–4.

PROTOTYPE: **Lichen amyloidosus**

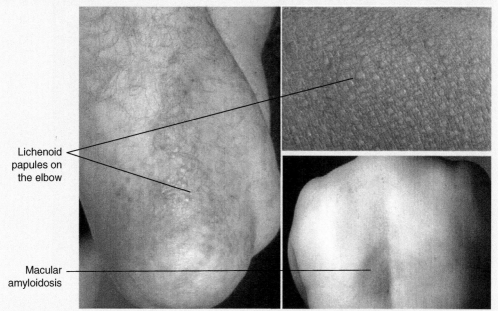

Lichenoid papules on the elbow

Macular amyloidosis

CI: Chronic and pruritic disease, showing firm, densely arranged papules with a lichenoid surface mostly on the extensor aspect of the extremities.

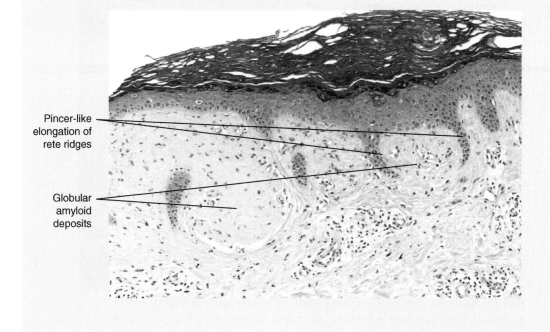

Pincer-like elongation of rete ridges

Globular amyloid deposits

DEPOSITION AND STORAGE

Lichen amyloidosus

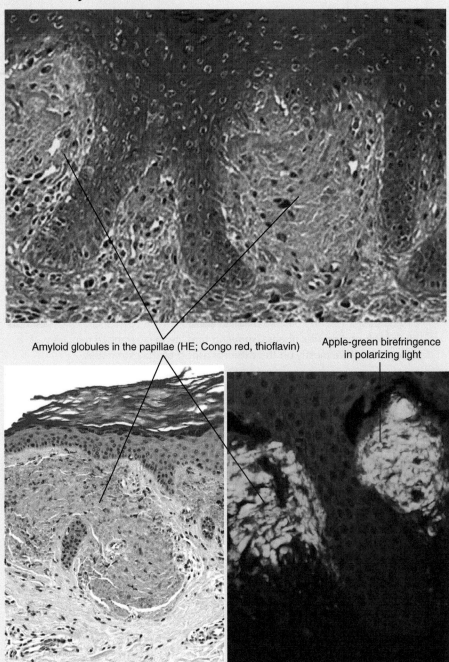

Amyloid globules in the papillae (HE; Congo red, thioflavin)

Apple-green birefringence in polarizing light

Hi: Eosinophilic globular deposits in the papillary dermis; expanding of dermal papillae by large clumps of amyloid in late stages; thinning of rete ridges; acanthosis, hyperkeratosis and hypergranulosis. Amyloid deposits are highlighted by apple-green birefringence under polarizing light in Congo-red or thioflavin stained specimens.

DIFFERENTIAL DIAGNOSIS: **Colloid milium**

Faint yellowish papules and plaques

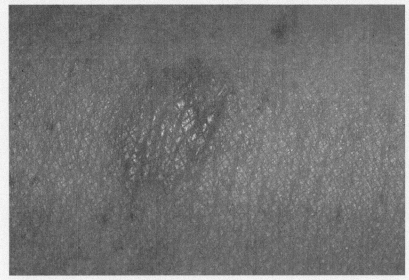

Cl: Yellowish tiny papules or plaques, in light exposed areas.

Clumped elastotic collagen

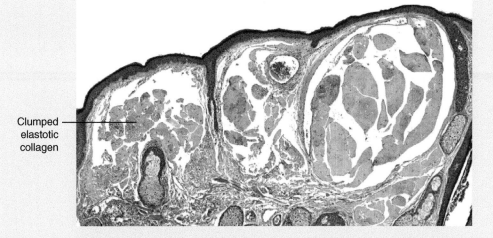

Hi: Globules of elastotic-staining degenerative collagen material in the upper and papillary dermis.

Other Diagnosis

Hyalinosis cutis et mucosae (lipoid proteinosis): Genetic disorder with accumulation of glycoproteins affecting skin, nervous system and other organs. Dermal deposits of amorphous eosinophilic hyaline material (PAS positive) with concentric rings around vessel walls and eccrine glands.

References

Breathnach, S. M. (1988). "Amyloid and amyloidosis." *J Am Acad Dermatol* **18**(1 Pt 1): 1–16.

Molina-Ruiz, A. M., L. Cerroni, *et al.* (2013). "Cutaneous Deposits." *Am J Dermatopathol* **36**(1): 1–48.

PROTOTYPE: **Calcinosis cutis**

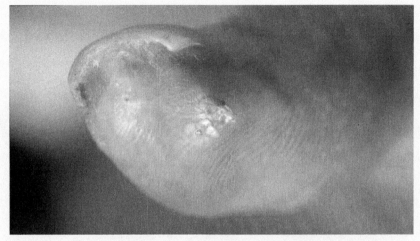

Calcinosis on
the tip of the
thumb

Cl: Various types of cutaneous calcification have to be differentiated:
metastatic, dystrophic and tumoral calcinosis, depending on the underlying
disorder and pathogenesis. Firm papules or subcutaneous plaques are found,
often with discharge of chalky material.

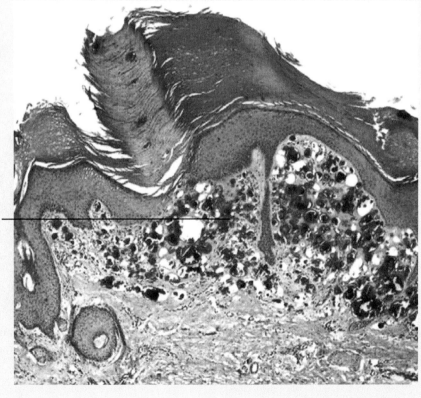

Calcium
deposits

Calcinosis cutis

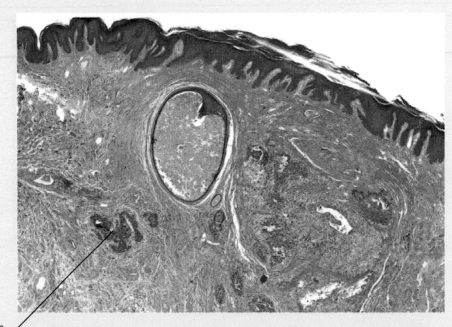

Calcium
deposits

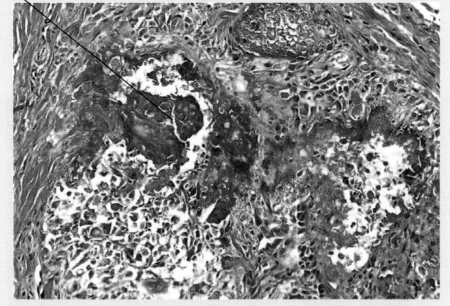

Hi: Crumbly, basophilic (H&E) masses in the dermis and/or subcutis, transepidermal elimination may be found, histiocytic and granulomatous foreign body reactions.

VARIANTS (depending on underlying disorder)

Dystrophic

Metastatic, D-hypervitaminosis, hyperparathyreoidism

Metabolic

Tumoral

Idiopathic

DEPOSITION AND STORAGE

DIFFERENTIAL DIAGNOSIS: **CREST-syndrome**

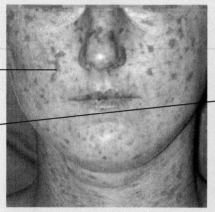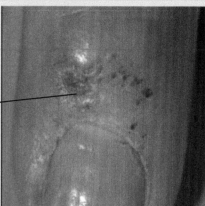

Telangiectasias in CREST - syndrome

Acral calcinosis in CREST - syndrome

Cl: Calcinosis, Raynaud syndrome, Esophageal involvement, systemic scleroderma, telangiectasias.

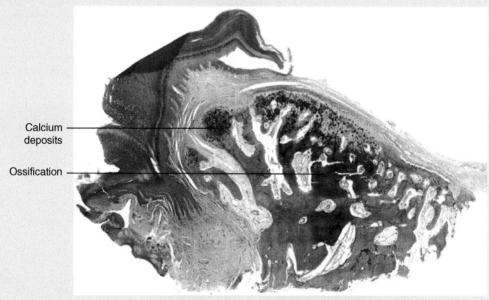

Calcium deposits

Ossification

Hi: Deposits of calcium in the upper dermis, transepidermal elimination, mixed cellular, occasionally granulomatous inflammatory infiltrate.

DIFFERENTIAL DIAGNOSIS: **Osteoma cutis, primary**

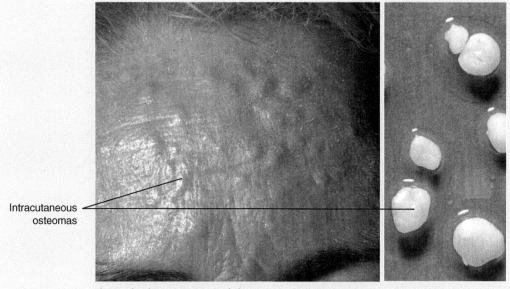

Intracutaneous osteomas

Cl: Hard subcutaneous nodules.

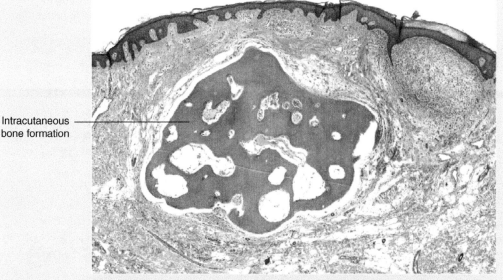

Intracutaneous bone formation

Hi: In the deep dermis or subcutis, lamellar ossification from condensed collagen, eosinophilic bone with formation of lacunae, osteoblasts embedded, inclusion of connective tissue with blood vessels (Haversian channels), osteoclasts and multinucleated giant cells in the periphery, hematopoiesis may be present.

Variant: *Albright's hereditary osteodystrophy: Ossification of condensed collagen (lamellar ossification); subungual exostosis: enchondral ossification with formation of mature trabecular bone.*

DEPOSITION AND STORAGE

DIFFERENTIAL DIAGNOSIS: **Tophus (gout)**

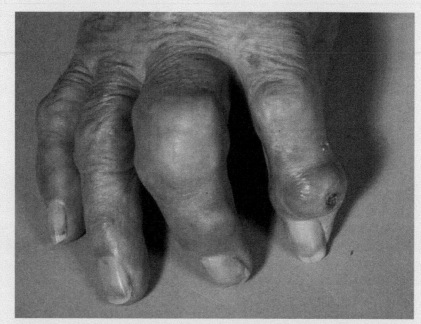

Ulcerated hard nodules

Cl: Accumulation of uric acid crystals in the subcutaneous tissue, presenting as nodules at digital joints, elbows and other sites, due to abnormal purine metabolism.

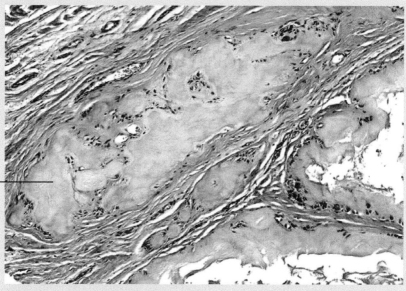

Amorphous and crystalline masses of mono-sodium urate monohydrate

Hi: Amorphous eosinophilic or greyish material in the dermis (crystals of sodium urate), needle like clefts, surrounded by palisading granuloma with foreign body giant cells. Fixation with formalin leaves empty spaces, whereas densely packed brown crystal needles with multicolor birefringence are seen when fixation with alcohol is used.

DIFFERENTIAL DIAGNOSIS: **Steroid deposits**

Scarring
atrophy

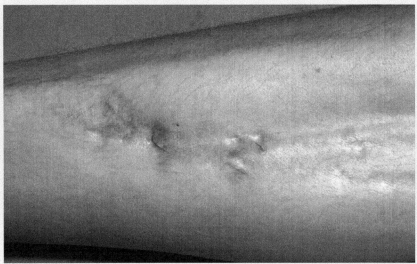

CI: Variable clinical presentation, often atrophy of the overlying epidermis and dermis.

Deposits of crystalline or
frothy material

Fibrosis

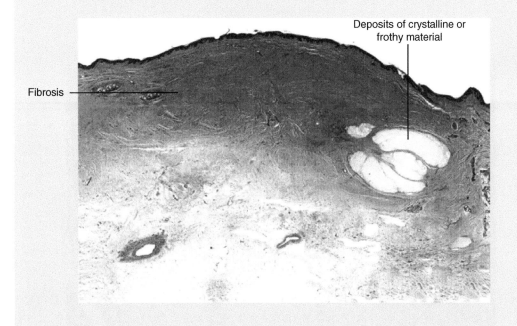

Steroid deposits

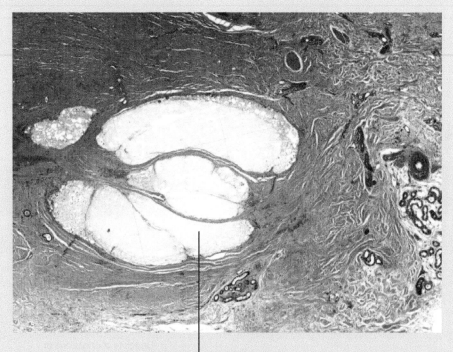

Deposits of frothy material

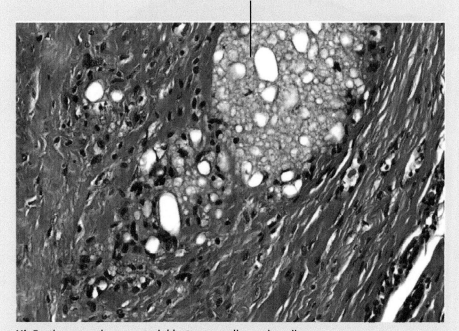

Hi: Frothy amorphous material between collagen bundles.

Other Diagnosis

Subcutaneous fat necrosis of newborn (adiponecrosis subcutanea neonatorum): exclusive subcutaneous localization, stellate clefting from triglyceride crystals, occasional calcification, spontaneous regression

Sclerema adiposum neonatorum (lethal)

Rheumatoid nodule (see Chapter 4, Granulomatous infiltrates, with necrosis, page 193*): Eosinophilic necrobiotic areas surrounded by palisading histiocytic infiltrate.*

Nevus of Nanta: Unna-type nevus with cutaneous ossification.

Calciphylaxis (see Chapter 5, Vasculopathic changes, page 261*)*

References

Abessi, B., D. R. Meyer, *et al.* (2012). "Osteoma cutis (nevus of nanta) of the eyebrow." *Ophthal Plast Reconstr Surg* **28**(1): 74–5.

Boyd, A. S. (2011). "Panniculitis ossificans traumatica of the lower leg." *Am J Dermatopathol* **33**(8): 858–60.

Cottoni, F., C. Dell' Orbo, *et al.* (1993). "Primary osteoma cutis. Clinical, morphological, and ultrastructural study." *Am J Dermatopathol* **15**(1): 77–81.

Eng, A. M. and E. Mandrea (1981). "Perforating calcinosis cutis presenting as milia." *J Cutan Pathol* **8**(3): 247–50.

Eulderink, F. and T. Postma (1997). "Demonstration of urate in formalin fixative as support for the histopathological diagnosis of gout." *Histopathology* **30**(2): 195.

Falasca, G. F. (2006). "Metabolic diseases: gout." *Clin Dermatol* **24**(6): 498–508.

Falsey, R. R. and L. Ackerman (2013). "Eruptive, hard cutaneous nodules in a 61-year-old woman.

Osteoma cutis in a patient with Albright hereditary osteodystrophy (AHO)." *JAMA Dermatol* **149**(8): 975–6.

Fernandez-Flores, A. (2011). "Calcinosis cutis: critical review." *Acta Dermatovenerol Croat* **19**(1): 43–50.

Gfesser, M., W. I. Worret, *et al.* (1998). "Multiple primary osteoma cutis." *Arch Dermatol* **134**(5): 641–3.

Haro, R., J. M. Revelles, *et al.* (2009). "Plaque-like osteoma cutis with transepidermal elimination." *J Cutan Pathol* **36**(5): 591–3.

King, D. F. and L. A. King (1982). "The appropriate processing of tophi for microscopy." *Am J Dermatopathol* **4**(3): 239.

Pugashetti, R., K. Shinkai, *et al.* (2011). "Calcium may preferentially deposit in areas of elastic tissue damage." *J Am Acad Dermatol* **64**(2): 296–301.

Reiter, N., L. El-Shabrawi, *et al.* (2011). "Calcinosis cutis: part I. Diagnostic pathway." *J Am Acad Dermatol* **65**(1): 1–12; quiz 13–14.

Samaniego-Gonzalez, E., A. Crespo-Erchiga, *et al.* (2009). "Perforans multiple osteoma cutis on the leg in a young woman." *J Cutan Pathol* **36**(4): 497–8.

Senti, G., M. H. Schmid, *et al.* (2001). "[Multiple miliary osteomata cutis. Excision with 'front lift' approach]." Hautarzt **52**(6): 522–5.

Talsania, N., V. Jolliffe, *et al.* (2011). "Platelike osteoma cutis." *J Am Acad Dermatol* **64**(3): 613–15.

Touart, D. M. and P. Sau (1998). "Cutaneous deposition diseases. Part I." *J Am Acad Dermatol* **39**(2 Pt 1): 149–71; quiz 172–4.

Touart, D. M. and P. Sau (1998). "Cutaneous deposition diseases. Part II." *J Am Acad Dermatol* **39**(4 Pt 1): 527–44; quiz 545–6.

CHAPTER 8

Adnexae

Atlas of Dermatopathology: Practical Differential Diagnosis by Clinicopathologic Pattern, First Edition.
Edited by Günter Burg MD, Werner Kempf MD, and Heinz Kutzner MD. Co-Editors: Josef Feit MD, and Laszlo Karai MD.
© 2015 John Wiley & Sons, Ltd. Published 2015 by John Wiley & Sons, Ltd.

PROTOTYPE: **Acne vulgaris**

Cl: Preferentially in younger age, in contrast to rosacea. During puberty very common disorder of variable form (see variants) and various degree.

Hi: The pilosebaceous unit is involved. Compact hyperkeratosis in the follicular infundibulum and cystic dilatation. Perifollicular mostly granulocytic inflammation and abscess formation of various degree depending on the form of acne. Scar formation in acne conglobata.

ADNEXAE

VARIANT: **Acne comedonica, Acne cystica**

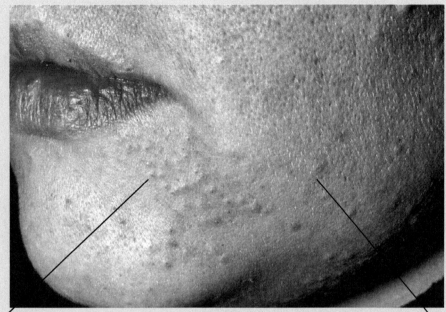

CI: Closed (whiteheads) comedos developing into open (blackheads) comedos.

Comedos

Cyst

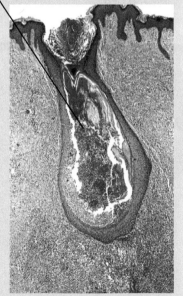

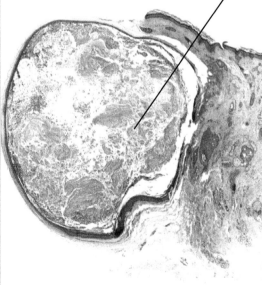

Hi: Dilated acroinfundibulum, filled with horn material, sebum, bacteria and debris (left). "Pseudocystic" structures derived from the infundibulum, filled with corneocytes, sebum, bacteria and debris (right).

VARIANT: Acne pustulosa

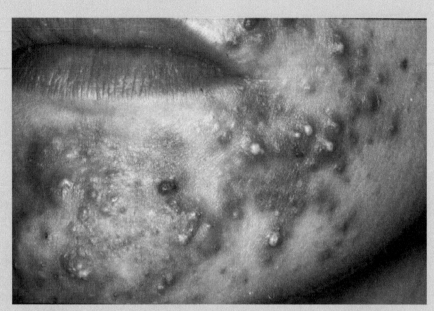

Inflammation
and pustules

Cl: Pustules.

Inflammatory infiltrate with
foreign body giant cells

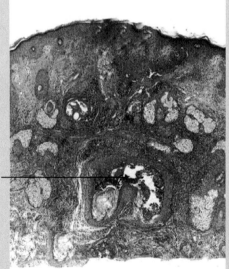

Destruction
of follicular
structures

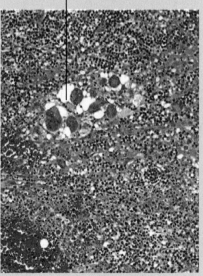

Hi: Mixed cellular, inflammatory infiltrate, due to foreign body and immunologic reactions.

Acne conglobata: *Severe form of acne.*
Acne fulminans: *Rare, severe, inflammatory, hemorrhagic and ulcerating variant of acne, involving predominantly chest and back.*
Acne inversa ("hidradenitis suppurativa").

PROTOTYPE: **Rosacea**

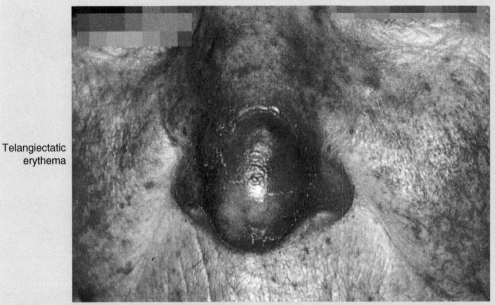

Telangiectatic erythema

Cl: Central face and cheeks, preferentially women: erythema, telangiectasias, papules and pustules.

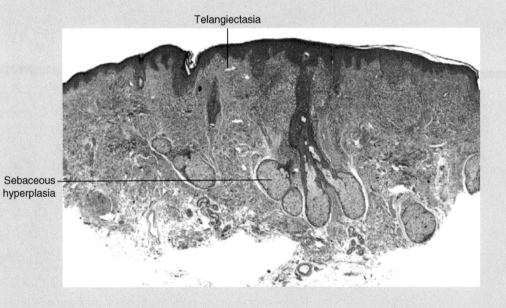

Telangiectasia

Sebaceous hyperplasia

Rosacea

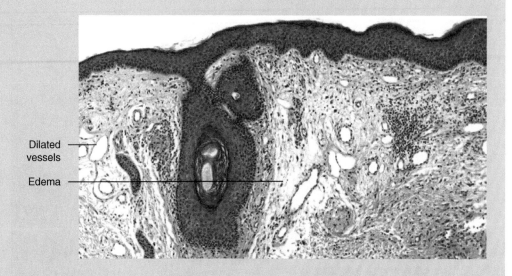

Dilated vessels

Edema

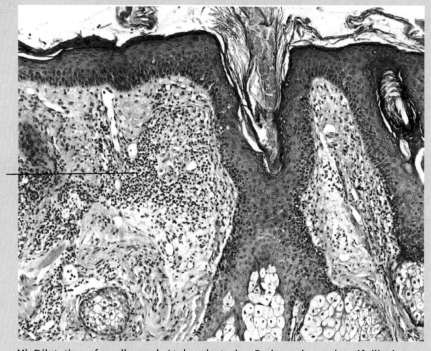

Lympho-histiocytic infiltrate with admixture of neutrophils and a few plasma cells

Hi: Dilatation of small vessels / telangiectasias. Perivascular and perifollicular lymphoid infiltrate, dermal edema, occasionally neutrophils and plasma cells, sebaceous hyperplasia.

VARIANT: Rosacea fulminans
(Synonym: Pyoderma faciale)

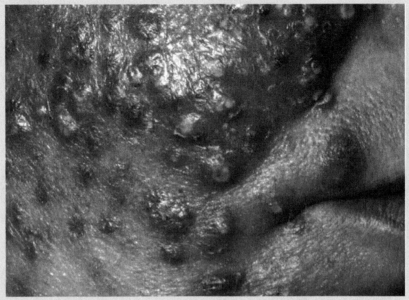

Pustules, inflammation

Cl: Sudden development of erythema, plaques and pustular nodules without any signs of acne.

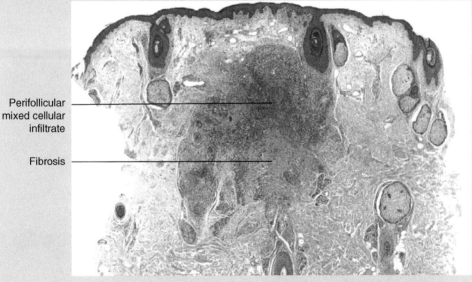

Perifollicular mixed cellular infiltrate

Fibrosis

Hi: Dense perivascular and perifollicular infiltrate, mostly eosinophils and neutrophils, occasionally plasma cells, infiltrate covering the whole dermis, septal and lobular panniculitis without leukocytoklasia.

ADNEXAE

VARIANT: **Rosacea, persistent edema (Morbihan)**

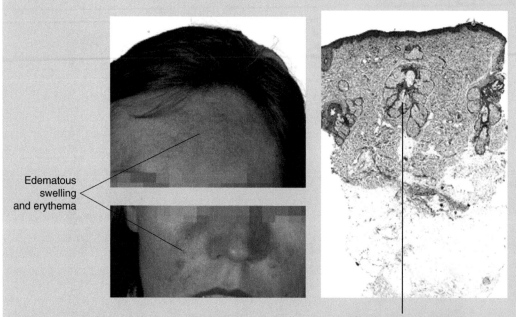

Edematous
swelling
and erythema

Sebaceous hyperplasia

Cl: Edematous swelling and erythema of the forehead and cheeks.

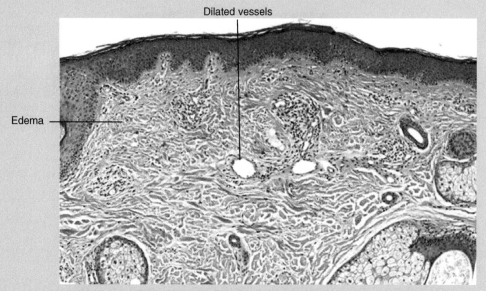

Dilated vessels

Edema

Hi: Overlapping features with rosacea, interstitial edema, telangiectasias, subtle perifollicular lymphohistiocytic infiltrate. Many dilated lymphatic vessels.

VARIANT: **Granulomatous rosacea**

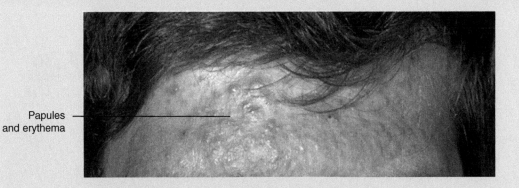

Papules
and erythema

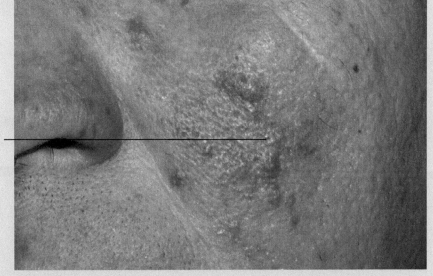

Papules
and erythema

Cl: Erythematous and slightly brownish plaques, papules or pustules in a
centrofacial distribution involving the forehead, nose and cheeks.

ADNEXAE

Granulomatous rosacea

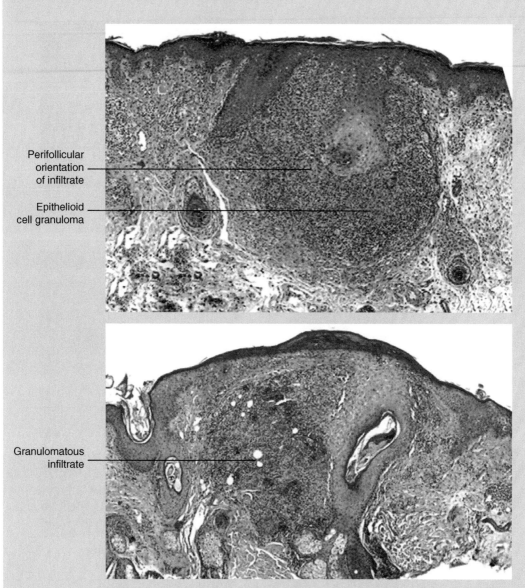

Perifollicular orientation of infiltrate

Epithelioid cell granuloma

Granulomatous infiltrate

Hi: Folliculocentric granulomatous dermal infiltrate with epithelioid cells and multinucleated giant cells of the Langhans-type, telangiectasias in the upper dermis, lymphocytes, neutrophils and plasma cells, sebaceous hyperplasia.

VARIANT: **Rosacea conglobata**

Nodular
abscesses

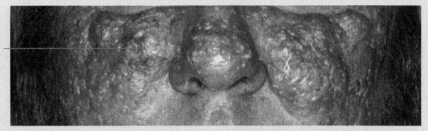

Cl: Severe form of rosacea, showing nodular abscess formation.

Abscess
formation

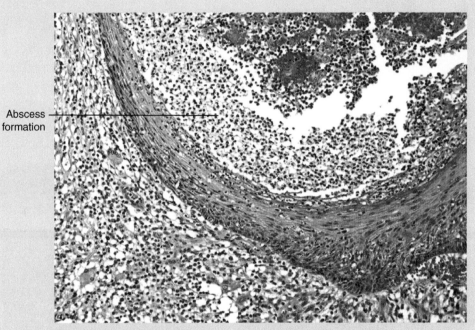

Hi: Extensive granulocytic infiltrate with massive damage of follicular structures and caseation necrosis.

ADNEXAE

PROTOTYPE: **Perioral dermatitis**

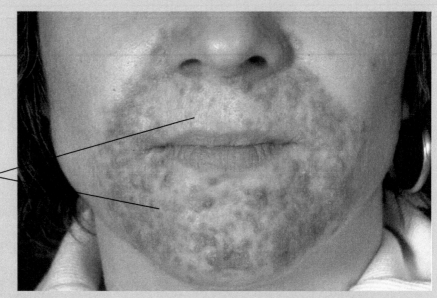

Papules
periorally,
sparing the
marginal zone

Cl: Younger patients with female preponderance, few or no telangiectasias.

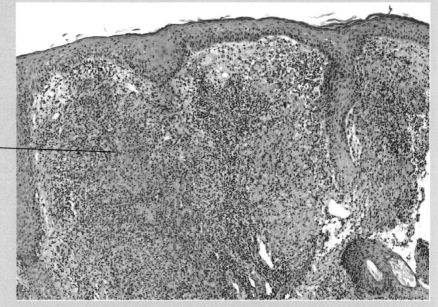

Lympho-
histiocytic
infiltrate

Hi: Lymphohistiocytic infiltrate, involving the hair follicle, granulomatous features may be present.

PROTOTYPE: **Rhinophyma**

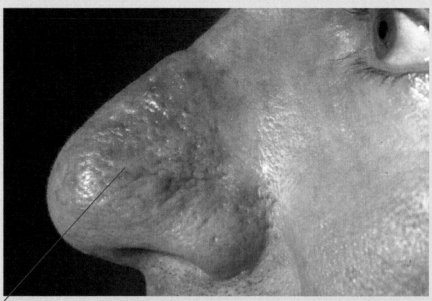

Cl: Disfiguring enlargement of the nose, oily skin, telangiectasias and prominent pores.

Sebaceous
hyperplasia

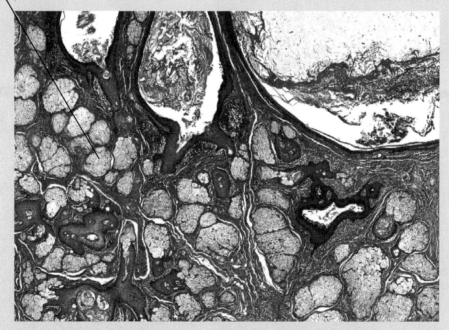

Hi: Extensive hyperplasia of sebaceous structures, telangiectasias, fibrosis.

ADNEXAE

DIFFERENTIAL DIAGNOSIS: Demodex folliculitis

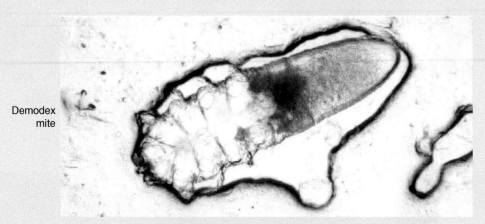

Demodex mite

Cl: Rosacea-like changes with papules and pustules, preferentially on the cheeks.

Demodex mites within the follicle

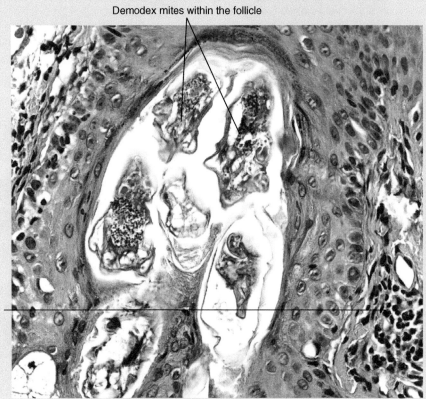

Lympho-histiocytic infiltrate with plasma cells

Hi: Demodex mites within the inflamed hair follicles with their heads towards the follicular opening; foreign-body reaction may be present.

ADNEXAE

DIFFERENTIAL DIAGNOSIS: *Pityrosporum* folliculitis

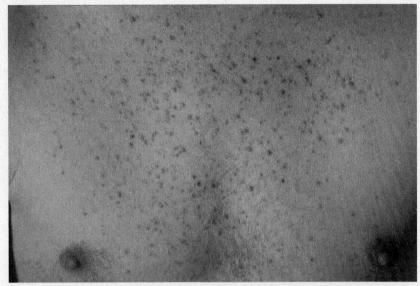

Tiny papules and pustules, follicle-bound

Cl: Acneiform reaction, preferentially involving the face, chest or back. Pruritus.

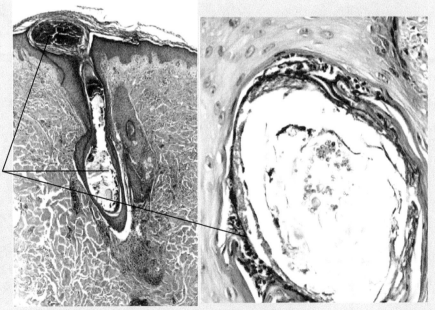

Detritus, hyperkeratotic material, mixed cellular infiltrate and spores in the follicles

Hi: Detection of spores within the inflamed hair follicles.

DIFFERENTIAL DIAGNOSIS: Bacterial folliculitis

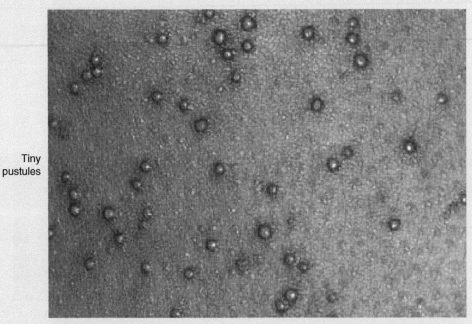

Tiny pustules

Cl: Acneiform reaction.

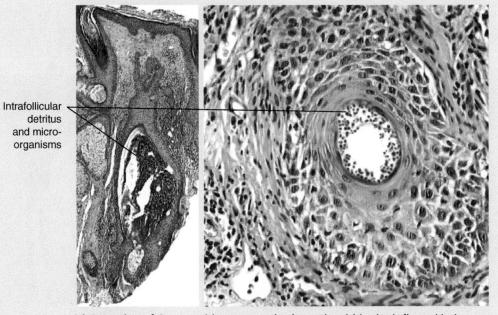

Intrafollicular detritus and micro- organisms

Hi: Detection of Gram positive or negative bacteria within the inflamed hair follicles, in the absence of demodex mites and *pityrosporum* spores.

DIFFERENTIAL DIAGNOSIS: Eosinophilic folliculitis and papular eruption of HIV

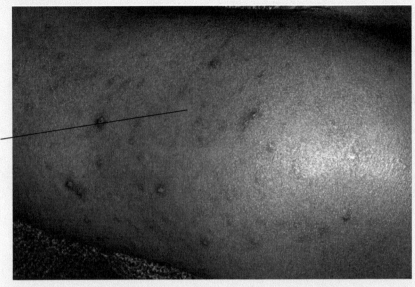

Tiny papules and pustules on the leg

Cl: Disseminated papules and pustules.

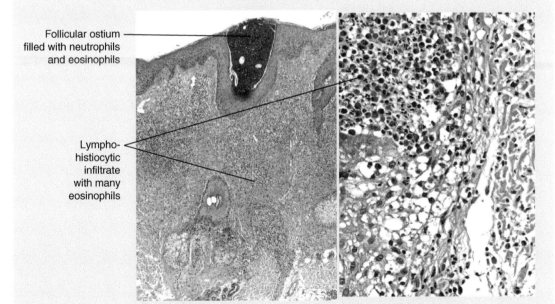

Follicular ostium filled with neutrophils and eosinophils

Lympho-histiocytic infiltrate with many eosinophils

Hi: Inflamed hair follicles with admixture of eosinophils; serological findings.

Trichophytia: Detection of hyphae in the inflamed hair follicle (PAS or Grocott stain).

Eosinophilic folliculitis Ofuji: Perifollicular lymphohistiocytic infiltrate with admixture of numerous eosinophils and accumulation of eosinophils in the ostia and infundibula of the inflamed hair follicles.

Lupus miliaris disseminatus faciei: Dermal granulomas with central necrosis and neutrophils (see Chapter 4, Granulomatous infiltrates, with necrosis, page 184).

References

Cribier, B. (2013). "Rosacea under the microscope: characteristic histological findings." *J Eur Acad Dermatol Venereol* **27**(11): 1336–43.

Perrigouard, C., B. Peltre, *et al.* (2013). "A histological and immunohistological study of vascular and inflammatory changes in rosacea." *Ann Dermatol Venereol* **140**(1): 21–9.

Sanchez, J. L., A. C. Berlingeri-Ramos, *et al.* (2008). "Granulomatous rosacea." *Am J Dermatopathol* **30**(1): 6–9.

ADNEXAE

PROTOTYPE: **Trichotillomania**

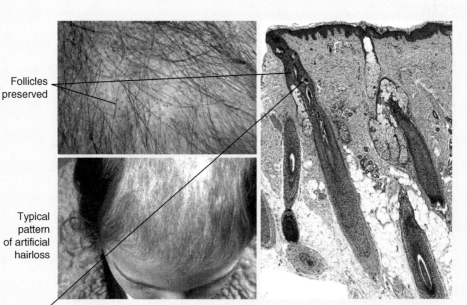

Follicles preserved

Typical pattern of artificial hairloss

Pigment casts

CI: Solitary, rarely multiple, circumscribed areas of incomplete hair loss with short hairs of varying length; only those hairs reaching at least 3 mm in length can be removed. The hair shafts often show distal splits and fringes. Broken-off hairs may appear as dark dots.

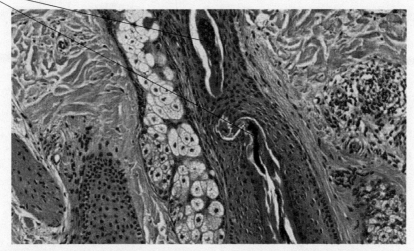

Hi: Normal epidermis, normal follicle counts, normal ratio of terminal to vellus hair, dilated, empty infundibuli, increased ratio of catagen and telogen hairs, clefts around the follicular epithelium, perifollicular erythrocytes and hemorrhage, no inflammatory infiltrate, trichomalacia may occur.

Variant: *Traction and pressure alopecia*

DIFFERENTIAL DIAGNOSIS: **Frontal fibrosing alopecia**

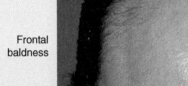

Frontal
baldness

Cl: Frontal baldness.

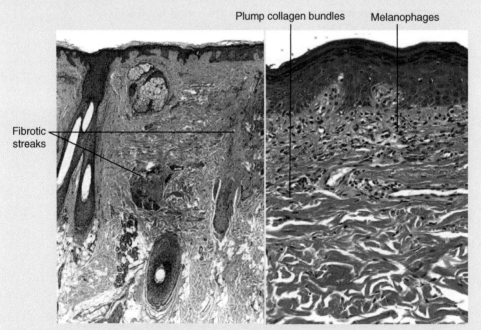

Plump collagen bundles   Melanophages

Fibrotic
streaks

Hi: Loss of hair follicles due to scarring process, variant of lichen planopilaris.

Comment
Frontal fibrosing alopecia is considered to be late stage lichen (ruber) planopilaris.

Alopecia areata (*see* Perifollicular inflammation, no fibrosis, page 342*).*

Androgenetic alopecia (*see* Perifollicular inflammation, no fibrosis, page 348): *Decreased ratio of vellus to terminal hairs, perifollicular lymphoid infiltrate often present, no trichomalacia.*

Diffuse telogen effluvium.

References

Davis-Daneshfar, A. and R. M. Trueb (1995). "[Tonsural trichotillomania]." *Hautarzt* **46**(11): 804–7.

Stefanato, C. M. (2010). "Histopathology of alopecia: a clinicopathological approach to diagnosis." *Histopathology* **56**(1): 24–38.

PROTOTYPE: **Alopecia areata**

ADNEXAE

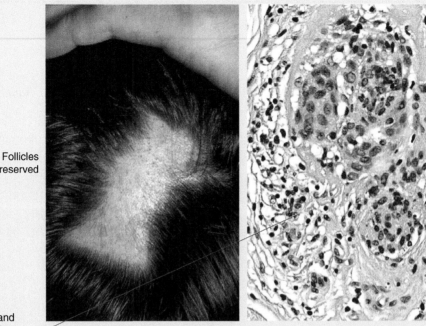

Follicles preserved

Peribulbar and intrabulbar lymphocytic infiltrate

Cl: Focal, multiple or diffuse non-inflamed, non-scarring process; can progress to loss of all scalp hairs (alopecia totalis) or all scalp and body hairs (alopecia universalis), sometimes associated nail changes (pitted nails).

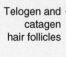

Telogen and catagen hair follicles

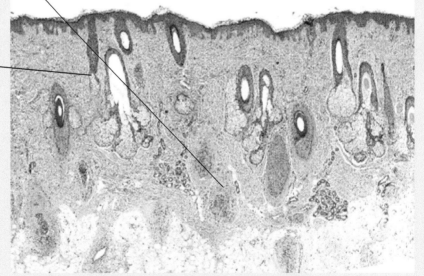

Hi: Peribulbar and intrabulbar lymphocytic infiltrate, decreased number of terminal anagen hairs, increased number of terminal catagen and telogen hairs, occasionally eosinophils, edema of hair matrix, pigment incontinence of hair bulbs, angiofibrotic strands.

VARIANT

Late stage: No or little perivascular or peribulbar infiltrates, increased number of miniaturized vellus hairs.

ADNEXAE

DIFFERENTIAL DIAGNOSIS: **Androgenetic alopecia**

Frontal
thinning
of hair

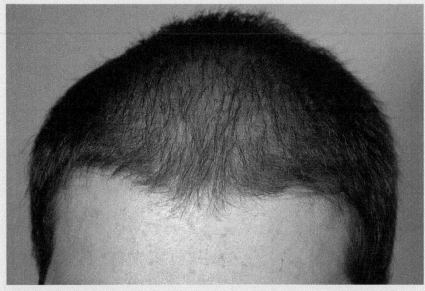

Cl: Diffuse hair loss, usually starting in the frontoparietal area; male or female pattern.

Vellus hair follicle

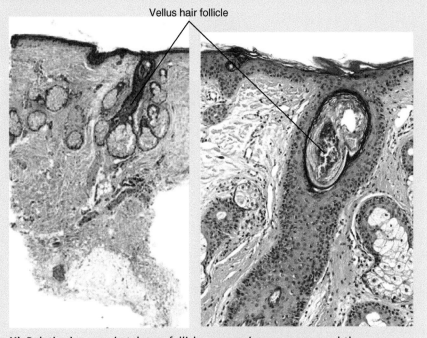

Hi: Relative increase in telogen follicles, no scaring, no or very subtle perifollicular inflammation.

Other Diagnosis

Frontal fibrosing alopecia (*see* No inflammation, no fibrosis, page 344).

Alopecia syphilitica (areolaris).

References

Ihm, C. W., S. S. Hong, *et al.* (2004). "Histopathological pictures of the initial changes of the hair bulbs in alopecia areata." *Am J Dermatopathol* **26**(3): 249–53.

Lee, J. Y. and M. L. Hsu (1991). "Alopecia syphilitica, a simulator of alopecia areata: histopathology and differential diagnosis." *J Cutan Pathol* **18**(2): 87–92.

Miteva, M., C. Misciali, *et al.* (2012). "Histopathologic features of alopecia areata incognito: A review of 46 cases." *J Cutan Pathol* **39**(6): 596–602.

Muller, C. S. and L. El Shabrawi-Caelen (2011). "'Follicular Swiss cheese' pattern – another histopathologic clue to alopecia areata." *J Cutan Pathol* **38**(2): 185–9.

Stefanato, C. M. (2010). "Histopathology of alopecia: a clinicopathological approach to diagnosis." *Histopathology* **56**(1): 24–38.

ADNEXAE

ADNEXAE

PROTOTYPE: Scarring alopecia, late stage (pseudopelade Brocq)

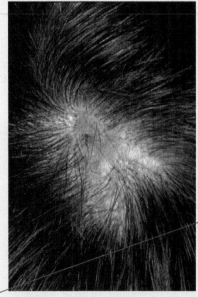
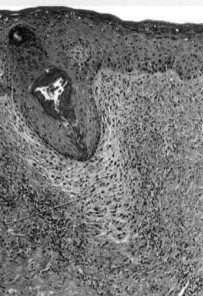

Follicles
lost

Scarring
of follicles

Cl: Like in alopecia areata, in "pseudo alopecia areata" there are small areas of alopecia without any scaring or significant inflammation. Some if not all cases possibly are late stages of either lupus erythematosus or lichen planus of the scalp.

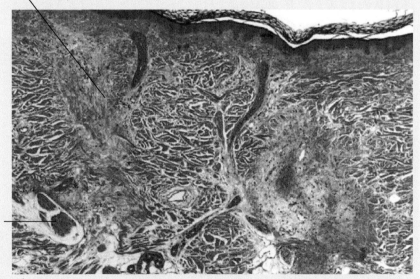

Remnants
of musculi
arrectores
pilorum

Hi: Follicular epithelial atrophy, concentric lamellar fibroplasias, foreign-body inflammation, selective loss of hair follicles and sebaceous glands, subtle perifollicular lymphohistiocytic infiltrate, epidermis normal or atrophic; fibrotic streaks.

VARIANTS

Early stage lichen ruber planopilaris: Lichenoid interface dermatitis, decreased number of follicles, no mucin deposits, perifollicular lymphocytic infiltrates, perifollicular fibroplasia.

Frontal fibrosing alopecia (*see* No inflammation, no fibrosis, page 344) is considered a variant of lichen (ruber) planopilaris.

ADNEXAE

DIFFERENTIAL DIAGNOSIS: Discoid lupus erythematosus, end stage

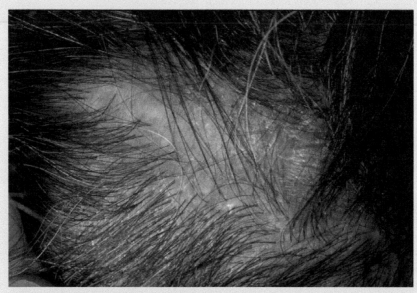

Cl: Scarring alopecia without follicles.

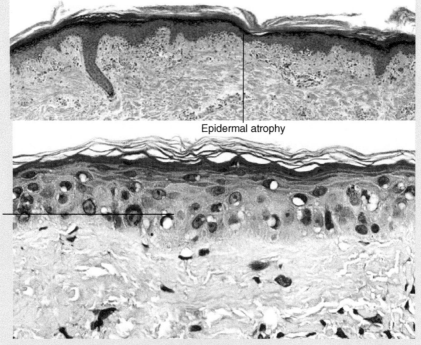

Epidermal atrophy

Damage of epidermal architecture

Hi: Atrophy, loss of follicular structures, fibrosis.

References

Annessi, G., G. Lombardo, *et al.* (1999). "A clinicopathologic study of scarring alopecia due to lichen planus: comparison with scarring alopecia in discoid lupus erythematosus and pseudopelade." *Am J Dermatopathol* **21**(4): 324–31.

Bergner, T. and O. Braun-Falco (1991). "Pseudopelade of Brocq." *J Am Acad Dermatol* **25**(5 Pt 1): 865–6.

Braun-Falco, O., S. Imai, *et al.* (1986). "Pseudopelade of Brocq." *Dermatologica* **172**(1): 18–23.

Moure, E. R., R. Romiti, *et al.* (2008). "Primary cicatricial alopecias: a review of histopathologic findings in 38 patients from a clinical university hospital in Sao Paulo, Brazil." *Clinics (Sao Paulo)* **63**(6): 747–52.

Silvers, D. N., B. E. Katz, *et al.* (1993). "Pseudopelade of Brocq is lichen planopilaris: report of four cases that support this nosology." *Cutis* **51**(2): 99–105.

Stefanato, C. M. (2010). "Histopathology of alopecia: a clinicopathological approach to diagnosis." *Histopathology* **56**(1): 24–38.

Trachsler, S. and R. M. Trueb (2005). "Value of direct immunofluorescence for differential diagnosis of cicatricial alopecia." *Dermatology* **211**(2): 98–102.

Whiting, D. A. (1999). "Traumatic alopecia." *Int J Dermatol* **38 Suppl 1**: 34–44.

ADNEXAE

Index

Note: Page numbers in *italics* refer to Figures.

Atlas of Dermatopathology: Practical Differential Diagnosis by Clinicopathologic Pattern, First Edition.
Edited by Günter Burg MD, Werner Kempf MD, and Heinz Kutzner MD. Co-Editors: Josef Feit MD, and Laszlo Karai MD.
© 2015 John Wiley & Sons, Ltd. Published 2015 by John Wiley & Sons, Ltd.